# PRAISE FOR *UNFINISHED BUSINESS*

For those entering or embracing their senior years, *Unfinished Business* is a must-read—a no-excuse blueprint that reignites purpose, power, and possibility amid the myths of inevitable decline. As a functional medicine practitioner, I applaud Dean's own health journey, which resonates with deep authenticity throughout the book.

Dean's guide delivers doable practical tools: mindset shifts for late starters, corrective exercises and nutrition for building mobility and endurance, and more. It rejects the status quo, empowering readers over 60 to shout "Not yet!" and claim their unfinished stories.

Dean's numerous certifications make him highly qualified to write this book, but it's his personal health transformation and engaging storytelling that will inspire you to take action for your own journey. This book belongs in the hands of everyone over 50!

**—Dr. Tonya Hartig, Ph.D.**
Doctor of Functional Medicine
The Well Being

This isn't another "feel-good" book about aging gracefully. It's a wake-up call wrapped in hope. Dean challenges the lies society tells us about getting older and replaces them with truth: you're not done, you're just getting started.

If you've ever wondered whether your best years are behind you, this book will remind you that your most impactful, purpose-filled years can still be ahead.

**—Michelle Cunningham**
International Bestselling Author, *Do It Anyway Girl*

As a lifelong educator, I've witnessed how powerful continued learning and self-discovery can be at every stage of life. In *Unfinished Business*, Dean Walters delivers a message that transcends age—one of courage, renewal, and personal accountability. He reminds us that growth doesn't stop with retirement or adversity; it begins again when we choose to take ownership of our health, our mindset, and our purpose.

Through stories, science, and simple truths, this book challenges older adults to see aging not as a season of decline, but as an extraordinary opportunity to build strength, resilience, and meaning. Dean's voice is authentic, practical, and deeply inspiring—a guide for anyone who believes their best work, and their greatest impact, may still lie ahead.

**—Larry W. Tyree, Ed.D.**
Professor Emeritus, University of Florida
President Emeritus, Gulf Coast State College,
Santa Fe College, College of the Florida Keys,
and Independence (KS) Community College

Dean Walters flips the script on aging. *Unfinished Business* isn't about slowing down—it's about rising up with renewed purpose, power, and possibility. A must-read for anyone who knows their best years are still ahead.

**—Sarah Robbins**
*USA Today* #1 Best Selling Author

# UNFINISHED BUSINESS

***The No-Excuse Blueprint for Aging with Purpose, Power, and Possibilities***

DEAN WALTERS

Unfinished Business

*The No-Excuse Blueprint for Aging with Purpose, Power, and Possibilities*



Aging Boldly
1745 Jefferson Ave.
Fort Myers, FL 33901
agingboldly.life

ISBN: 979-8-9931662-6-1

Book Design by Transcendent Publishing
Editing by Mary Rembert

***Medical Disclaimer***

This book is for informational and educational purposes only. It is not intended to provide, and should not be construed as, medical advice. I am not a physician or a licensed physical therapist, and I do not diagnose, treat, or prescribe for medical conditions.

I am a Certified Integrative Nutrition Health Coach and certified in senior fitness, corrective exercise, and fitness nutrition. I am trained to help individuals use exercise to improve mobility, strength, and overall wellness, as well as to address lifestyle factors that may impact health, such as stress management, nutrition, and daily habits. While I am not a licensed clinical nutritionist, I may offer general information about food and nutrition that has been helpful to others.

Always consult with your physician or qualified healthcare provider before beginning any new exercise, nutrition, or wellness program. Your health and safety are ultimately your responsibility.

*"Master your age, master your life."*

–Dean Walters

# CONTENTS

# DEDICATION

This book is dedicated to the following:

For every person over 60 who was told, “Just slow down,” but didn’t.

For those who’ve buried parts of themselves … dreams, purpose, energy … and are digging them back up.

For those who ache when they move, but move anyway.

For those who feel invisible in a world that stopped seeing them, but are ready to be seen again.

For those who’ve been told their thoughts didn’t matter, their opinions were outdated, their voice was no longer needed, but knew, deep down, they still had something to say.

For the ones who have sat in too many waiting rooms and heard too many diagnoses, but decided *that’s not how my story ends.*

For those who’ve been told, “It’s just getting older,” but knew there had to be a better answer.

For those who’ve cared for others their whole lives, and are finally ready to care for themselves.

For those who’ve lost a step, but not their spark.

For those who want to climb stairs, not stare at them.

For those who’ve been knocked down by pain, loss, fear, or failure, but got back up, even if it took everything they had.

For the man wondering if his strength will ever return.

For the woman asking if her best years are already behind her.

For the ones who’ve spent too long feeling unheard, underestimated, or left behind.

For anyone who has ever whispered, “Is this it?” and is ready to shout, “Not yet!”

This is your call to rise!

You’re not done.

You’re just getting started.

You’ve got **unfinished business.**

And this time … **you’re not doing it alone.**

# FOREWORD

**By Forbes Riley**

Power. Choice. Action.

These three words separate dreamers from doers—and Dean Walters is a doer.

When I first encountered Dean's message, I felt it in my gut. This isn't another motivational pep talk or feel-good success manual. This book is a wake-up call; a call to *own your story*, *get off the sidelines*, and *refuse to let age, fear, or excuses define your future.*

As someone who's reinvented myself more times than I can count—from actress to entrepreneur, from TV host to the "Queen of Pitch"—I know the truth Dean is sharing here: it's never too late to take control of your life. The moment you stop waiting for permission, everything changes.

Dean doesn't just teach theory; he *lives* what he writes. Every chapter of this book carries the heartbeat of experience, resilience, and grit. He reminds us that the only thing standing between where you are and where you want to be is the story you keep telling yourself, and he hands you the tools to rewrite it.

So, here's my challenge to you: don't just read this book. *Use it.* Let Dean's words push you, stretch you, and remind you that it's not time that's running out—it's belief that needs to catch up.

Because your next chapter doesn't start when the world gives you permission.

It starts the moment you decide to turn the page.

With admiration,
**Forbes Riley**
International Speaker & Visionary Entrepreneur
Award-Winning TV Host & Master of the Pitch

# PREFACE

Let's get one thing straight: aging isn't the slow crawl to the grave you've been sold. It's not the steady decline the doctors warn you about. And it sure as hell isn't a life sentence to weakness, pain, and invisibility.

I know. I've been there.

I've stared down illness, accidents, surgeries, and setbacks that nearly broke me.

Sixteen years ago, I could have easily bought the story that "this is just how it goes" after a certain age. Instead, I rebuilt my body, my health, and my life from the ground up. And I discovered something the medical world doesn't like to admit: most of us are capable of 10 times more strength, healing, and vitality than we've been led to believe.

Who am I? Why would you listen to what I have to say?

I'm a Certified Integrative Nutrition Health Coach. I hold six certifications from the International Sports Science Association—Senior Fitness, Corrective Exercise, Fitness Nutrition, and more.

I've trained specifically in exercises for knee and hip replacement recovery, shoulder stabilization, Parkinson's disease, breast cancer survivorship, and the physiology of obesity. That's hard-won expertise that I've used to help hundreds of older adults stop surrendering and start living again.

But let me be blunt: I'm angry (pissed, really).

Angry at a system that doles out pills faster than it doles out hope.

Angry at the quiet message society sends that after 60, your job is to shrink, fade, and wait.

Angry at the number of people who accept decline as destiny.

Every time I turn on the TV, I see another commercial about the extra benefits we need from Medicare: the latest new medication for things that hardly existed 30 years ago, a new hearing aid, walk-in showers, upright walkers, adult diapers, cremations, funeral insurance, and on and on and on.

As we get older, our views and wisdom are no longer valued. We become invisible and mark time until we end up an invalid waiting for the obituary to be written. IT DOESN'T HAVE TO BE THIS WAY!

We've all seen posts on social media about the 90-year-old yoga teacher, or the 82-year-old man who just set a world record in the senior Olympics, or the grandmother who wrestled a would-be thief to the ground until police arrived.

As inspiring as those stories are, let's face it … they're the unicorns of aging, the exceptions, if you will, and the rest of us are the rule!

This book is for all of us who may never set a world record for a senior anything, except possibly snoring. It is for all of us who have lived a full but hard life and are ready to enjoy its rewards. Rewards, though, can be difficult to enjoy if we don't have our health.

This book is for all of us who bear the battle scars of life—the injuries, the diseases, the genetics, or the bad choices that have brought us to a state of *dis*-ease.

We may have lost an inch or two in height over the years, and we may have put on some weight. We probably can't bend as far, jump as high, lift as much, or sleep as well.

But we're not ready to quit. We want to change where we are now to where we want to be—healthier, more rested, more flexible, stronger, more alert, more relaxed, more energetic, more relevant ... basically, happier!

What I've seen—what I've lived—is a generation slowly backing away from the life they still want and still deserve.

I wrote this book because I believe that narrative has to change. This isn't about chasing youth; it's about reclaiming ownership. Of our health. Our strength. Our voice. Our impact.

You'll see stories on the following pages. Some are about me; others are about friends or clients (shared with their permission, of course). Many will likely echo your own story. But more than stories, you'll find a blueprint.

This book is not a pat on the back or a gentle nudge. It's a wake-up call—one that isn't coddling or complicated, but a clear and doable battle plan for reclaiming your strength, your purpose, and your power.

If you're ready to stop making excuses, stop settling, and stop living smaller than you were meant to—then keep reading.

You don't need to be perfect. You just need to start.

Because you and I? We still have **unfinished business**.

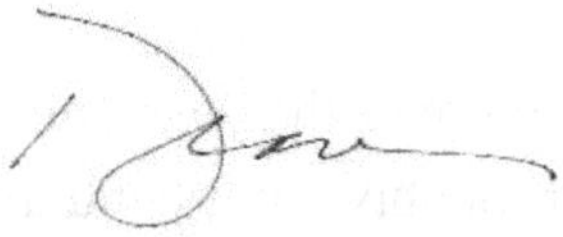

# INTRODUCTION

*"Most people don't age. They surrender."*

–Dean Walters

If you're holding this book, you probably know what I mean. You've seen the slow fade: less movement, more meds, shrinking goals, expanding waistlines, and an eerie sense that the world is politely forcing you toward the sidelines.

Not on my watch.

I wrote this book because I'm tired of seeing older adults being treated like they've already lived their best years. And I'm REALLY tired of seeing them act like it too. The truth is, we're not done yet.

We have **unfinished business**.

I know this personally. I've been through surgeries, injuries, and a radical career change. From opera houses to home gyms, I've reinvented myself—not because it was easy, but because not changing would have been fatal.

This isn't a feel-good guide full of platitudes. It's a *blueprint* for reclaiming control of your body, your mind, your movement, your joy, and your place in this world.

So … I'm calling you out. But I'm also here to walk alongside you.

Inside, you'll find:

- A no-excuse breakdown of what's really causing decline (hint: it's not just aging)
- Tools, habits, and mindset shifts that work, even if you're "starting late"
- Links to deeper resources, like my online programs and a community of people who are rewriting the second half of their story

I hope you'll be one of them.

Let's not go quietly. Let's go boldly.

You're not done.

You're just getting started.

You've got **unfinished business**.

## CHAPTER 1

# FLAT ON MY BACK

*"The tragedy of life is not that it ends so soon, but that we wait so long to begin it."*

–W.M. Lewis

I didn't feel powerful.
I didn't feel wise.
I didn't feel useful.
I didn't feel like a man with decades of experience.
Or a performer.
Or a husband.
Or even myself.

I felt invisible.
I felt ashamed.
I felt broken.

As I lay flat on my back in a hospital bed in the middle of our living room in the Florida Keys, I stared at the ceiling and kept asking one question: "What the hell am I going to do now?"

The quadriceps tendons in my legs had ruptured. The surgeries to reattach the shredded tendons and ligaments in *both* legs had been extensive, and the braces (those damned braces) stretched from my hips to my ankles, locking me in place like some kind of medieval armor.

The pain meds were wearing off. And the reality was setting in.

It was 2009. I was 58. And my life had just been ripped apart.

My aging parents, well into their own senior years, drove all the way down from Indiana to take care of *me* for seven weeks. Why? So my wife could keep working at her own business and keep a roof over our heads. Someone had to fix my meals, bathe me, dress me, and help me out of bed and in and out of the bathroom.

Let me tell you something about swallowing your pride: it goes down like broken glass.

Recovery is “simple,” at least on paper. You follow a physical therapy plan. You move, stretch, rebuild. Slowly. Consistently.

But no one tells you how to recover mentally.

No one prepares you for the anger, the embarrassment, the questions that show up at 3 a.m.

No one warns you about the moment you look down at your body and wonder, *Will I ever trust you again?*

No one talks about the guilt you feel when your wife has to carry the full responsibility load. Or the look in your parents’ eyes when they try to hide their worry behind a smile. Or the way your sense of identity quietly walks out the door … and doesn't come back.

And somewhere amidst the pain, the pills, and the silence, it hits you:

Your old "normal" is gone.

You're not going back to how things were.

The questions now become, "*What's next?*" and "*What will my life look like from here?*"

This was where my journey truly began. Not on the operating table, but in that still, heavy moment, flat on my back … when I made the decision that I wasn't going to stay there. I had performed opera and musical theatre all of my adult life, but those days were about to change.

That moment, flat on my back, staring at the ceiling, wasn't just a turning point in my recovery. It was a wake-up call.

And the truth is, *we all have one*.

A moment when we realize that life has changed.

Our bodies don't bounce back like they used to. Energy runs low. Pain hangs around longer. The mirror reflects differently.

Deep down, we know: The way things were will never be that way again.

That realization might come after a surgery like mine. Or after a diagnosis. Or a fall. Or the day you can't get up off the floor without help. Or when you suddenly need help opening jars, tying your shoes, or catching your breath at the top of the stairs.

These moments aren't just inconvenient; they are identity-shaking.

When you're faced with a choice:

You can give in.

You can let the decline settle in.

You can start shrinking your life to match your limitations.

Or …

You can fight.

You can dig deep.

You can make new decisions.

You can take control of the things you *can* control.

That's why I started my business, *Aging Boldly.* I never wanted to feel that dependent again, not if I had any say in the matter. I didn't want my story to end in a recliner, fading into the background, waiting for the next doctor visit or prescription refill.

I wanted to move again. I wanted to be strong again.

I decided not just to help myself, but to help others do the same.

This book is for every man or woman who's had *that* moment … who's felt the ground shift beneath them … and is ready to stop waiting and start *fighting* for what comes next.

Your story isn't over.

YOU get to decide how the next chapter goes.

### Three Key Takeaways

1. Responsibility is non-negotiable—no one is coming to save your health; it's on you.
2. Your past setbacks are not your limiters—they can actually become your motivation.
3. Complacency is the real enemy—decline is not inevitable unless you let it be.

### Three Discussion/Reflection Questions

1. Have you been waiting for someone else to "fix" your health instead of owning it yourself?
2. What past setback or illness has shaped your thinking about what's possible for you?
3. In what area of your life have you accepted decline as "just part of aging"?

### Three Action Steps

1. Write down your true, unfiltered feelings about your current state of health.
2. Reframe one of your setbacks into a sentence of motivation and possibility.
3. Declare one area where you refuse to settle for decline, and make it visible in your home.

Awareness is the first step in reclaiming your power.

You've got **unfinished business**. And I'm here to help you do it.

CHAPTER 2

# INVISIBILITY—THE DAY I REALIZED I WASN'T SEEN ANYMORE

*"You are never too old to set another goal or to dream a new dream."*

–C.S. Lewis

I was standing in line at the pharmacy. My back ached. My knees hurt. I'd been in rehearsals all week, pushing through. And when I stepped up to the counter, the young clerk barely looked at me.

No eye contact.

No acknowledgment.

They just scanned my items as if I were invisible.

Now, even though I used to perform for thousands of people in full costumes under thousand-watt lights, I'm not someone who needs applause at CVS.

But in that moment, at that counter, in front of someone not even old enough to legally drink, I felt like I'd disappeared.

Not just from the spotlight, but from society.

That was the day I realized that aging isn't just physical. It's emotional. And if we're not careful, we start fading long before we should.

For many of us, invisibility starts subtly:

- People stop asking for your opinion.
- You're passed over for opportunities—"it's time for the younger generation."
- You sit at the table, but no one really listens.

And the worst part? We start believing it.

We shrink our goals. Our presence. Our voice.

It's not just ageism from the outside. It's self-erasure from the inside.

## The Lie We've Been Sold

Aging isn't the problem. The real problem is what we've been *taught to believe about aging.*

Somewhere along the way, the world started whispering lies into our ears; so quietly, and so often, that we started believing them:

> "You're not supposed to feel great after 60."
>
> "Slow down."
>
> "Take it easy."
>
> "Let the younger folks handle it."

"Your time has passed."

"It's normal to be tired, stiff, and forgetful."

"This is just how it is now."

And before we knew it, we were shrinking our lives to fit someone else's idea of what getting older looks like.

We stopped reaching.

Stopped stretching.

Stopped showing up in rooms we used to own.

Here's the truth no one wants to say out loud: Much of what we call "aging" is just neglect.

And while it may not completely be your fault, *it is still your responsibility.*

We've been marketed pills instead of purpose, comfort instead of challenge, and resignation instead of resilience.

But here's what I know because I've lived it:

- When you move your body, it responds.
- When you feed it well, it thanks you.
- When you stretch, strengthen, and support it consistently, it starts showing up for you again.
- When you stop accepting decline as inevitable, you start aging *on your terms.*

That's the heart of this book.

This isn't a pep talk or a feel-good memoir. This is a blueprint.

Not to get back what was lost, but to build what's still possible.

You don't have to train like a 20-year-old.

You don't have to run marathons, give up chocolate, or live at the gym.

But you do have to stop believing the lie that aging is a downhill slide that you can't stop.

There is a difference between growing older and giving up.

## The Cost of Doing Nothing—Here's What Invisibility Breeds

### *Loneliness*

This isn't just about not having company over for dinner. It's about a profound, gnawing sense of disconnection that seeps into your soul.

Loneliness can actually change your physiology. Studies show it increases inflammation, raises cortisol (your stress hormone), and literally shortens your life expectancy on par with smoking a pack of cigarettes every day.

The problem is, it's not loud or dramatic. It's slow, quiet, and sneaky. It creeps in when you decline an invitation because "you're too tired." It deepens when you think, *I'll just stay home; it's easier.*

And the longer it stays, the more it convinces you that this is normal.

It's not.

We are hardwired for connection. Without it, we begin to vanish from our own lives.

### *Depression & Cognitive Decline*

The brain is a muscle of sorts. It thrives when it's challenged, engaged, and used.

Purpose is its fuel. When that purpose is stripped away by retirement, loss, physical limitations, or being overlooked, the brain starts idling in neutral.

Memory falters.

Creativity dulls.

Motivation evaporates.

Depression often slips in, many times disguised as "just being tired" or "slowing down."

And here's the hard truth: when your mind isn't being fed new challenges and meaningful work, it starts shutting down parts of itself that aren't being used.

That's why engagement, whether through learning, volunteering, teaching, or creating, isn't optional for healthy aging. It's medicine.

### *Physical Deterioration*

Social interaction and physical movement are deeply linked. When you get out, you move more; whether that's walking from the parking lot, standing to greet someone, or dancing at a party.

When you stop showing up, your world shrinks physically and literally.

Muscle mass declines. Balance worsens. Endurance evaporates. Once you lose enough strength, even basic independence, like getting out of a chair, climbing stairs, or carrying groceries, becomes a challenge.

This is how people go from just "slowing down" to being fully dependent. Not because their bodies suddenly gave out, but because they stopped requiring their bodies to show up to do the work!

It's a slippery slope … from being overlooked … to feeling invisible … to believing you don't matter anymore.

And once you believe that you don't matter, you stop acting like you do.

That is the single most dangerous crossroad in the aging journey.

## The No-Excuse Blueprint to Becoming Visible Again

1. **Reclaim Your Voice.**

   Visibility starts with your words. It's tempting to stay quiet when you feel out of practice, you're worried about "saying the wrong thing," or you assume no one's interested. But silence only feeds invisibility.

   Start small. Ask someone how they're doing and listen like it matters because it does. Share a memory that fits the conversation. Give your opinion in a group, even if you feel a bit rusty.

The more you speak, the more you sharpen that skill. And the more you use your voice, the more others will listen.

You matter. Act like it.

2. **Move Toward the Light.**

   Isolation lives in the shadows, and the shadows grow larger when we stay still.

   Step into places where energy is moving: a fitness class, a choir, a hiking group, a book club, a painting workshop, or an online community like *Aging Mastery*. You can check out our community of your peers at https://info.agingboldly.life.

   This isn't just about "being seen." It's about surrounding yourself with life: with people, with laughter, with ideas, with movement.

   And here's the beautiful part: when you walk toward the light, you often end up *becoming* the light for someone else.

3. **Show Up Differently.**

   Your body sends messages about you before you even say a word.

   - A slouched posture says, *I'm trying not to be noticed.*
   - A flat expression says, *I'm done engaging.*
   - Neutral clothing says, *I'm just blending in.*

   Want to change the message?

   - Stand taller; it lifts your mood *and* makes you look more confident.

- Make eye contact; it tells people, *I see you.*
- Wear a splash of color; it says, *I'm alive and well.*
- Smile first; it opens doors before words even arrive.

Half of visibility is posture and presence. The other half? *Choosing* to bring energy into the room.

4. **Give Your Story Away.**

You've lived decades of life that someone else could benefit from *right now*. Wisdom wasted is wisdom lost.

- Mentor a younger colleague.
- Volunteer at a school or library.
- Record your family stories for your grandchildren.
- Write an article.
- Teach a skill.

When you give your story away, you're not giving up your relevance; you're multiplying it. Your story might be the spark someone else needs to light their own path.

5. **Change the Narrative.**

Every time you say, "I'm too old" or "It's not my time anymore," your mind files it away as truth, and your body acts accordingly.

Replace those phrases with "I'm just getting started" or "This is my time."

Your brain listens. Your energy listens. Your life listens.

Aging boldly starts in the way you speak about yourself.

**Three Key Takeaways**

1. Aging is not a slow decline—it's a stage of growth, purpose, and power.
2. Society's script is wrong—our culture may treat older adults as invisible, but you get to write your own story.
3. Your mindset determines your aging—whether you think your life matters, or you think it doesn't, you're right.

**Three Discussion Questions**

1. What story have you been told (or told yourself) about what aging looks like?
2. What things in your life have made you feel invisible, underestimated, or dismissed?
3. How could changing your perspective on aging change your daily choices?

**Three Action Steps**

1. Write a new personal definition of what your life should look like.
2. Identify one area of life where you've "shrunk back" and decide how you'll step forward again.
3. Create a simple mantra (e.g., *"I am not invisible. I have knowledge and experience to offer."*) and repeat it daily.

Being invisible isn't the problem.

Staying invisible is. Be louder. Be bolder.

Be the one who proves that purpose doesn't age out.

Because you've got **unfinished business**.

CHAPTER 3

# JOINT PAIN & IMMOBILITY—WHEN STIFFNESS FEELS LIKE A LIFE SENTENCE, NOT JUST A SYMPTOM

*"Those who think they have not time for bodily exercise will sooner or later have to find time for illness."*

–Edward Stanley

## The Day Her Keys Taught Her a Lesson

I've trained many people in their 60s and beyond, and each one has a specific story that convinced them to reach out to me. I gather stories from other coaches too, and this one fits right into the message in this book.

One client (let's call her Camille) was a retired ballet dancer. This is Camille's story.

**Coach:** (during the intake interview): *"So, Camille, what brought you to me today?"*

**Camille:** *"Well, I dropped my keys!"*

**Coach:** *"Uh ... you dropped your keys?"*

**Camille:** *"You don't understand. I wasn't doing yoga or dancing or even carrying an armload of groceries."*

**Coach:** *"OK?"*

**Camille:** *"I was just standing in my kitchen, thinking about lunch. My hand slipped. The keys dropped to the floor."*

**Coach:** *"OK?"*

**Camille:** *"I dropped my keys ... and there they stayed! I froze, staring down at them like they were a hundred miles away. I really wanted to pick them up, but I wasn't sure if I could. My knees started to hurt just thinking about it! And my lower back tensed like it was bracing for an earthquake!"*

(They both started to chuckle at the scene she created, but the coach realized, between chortles, that the little daily things we take for granted are the first ones to be taken away from us.)

**Coach:** *"So, what did you do then?"*

**Camille:** *"For a second, I just stood there ... thinking ... I could shuffle over to a chair, use it to lower myself down, grab the keys, and then hope I could get up without too much* *groaning ... or I could just leave them there and grab the spare set."*

**Coach:** *"Wow!"* (They both got a kick out of that, but then her mood shifted.)

**Camille:** *"But then I realized, those weren't just keys. It was an example of what was in store for me if I didn't do something. I didn't like what I saw."*

**Coach:** *"I get it, Camille, I get it! How long after that did you call me?"*

**Camille:** *"As soon as I finally managed to squat down and get those damned keys!"*

They chuckled again, and then he asked:

**Coach:** *"What are you willing to do so that doesn't happen again?"*

She looked at the coach and, without hesitation, said:

**Camille:** *"Anything, and everything. When do we start?"*

Camille is the best kind of client to work with—one who has stared into the mirror of what's in store for them, and decided to take their health back. And they always succeed!

You see, that moment wasn't just inconvenient for her; it was humiliating. But as much as it hurt, it was also clarifying. Her joints weren't broken; they were just ignored.

Like anything in life that gets ignored—relationships, skills, dreams—they start to shut down.

That was the day she realized that if she didn't change course, her body would start locking itself down for good.

## The Problem

Here's the brutal truth: **Motion is life.**

The second you stop moving, your body thinks it's a command: "I guess you don't need us anymore, so we'll just shut it down."

Our bodies are masters of efficiency. If you don't use something, your body shifts the energy somewhere else.

- Stop challenging your muscles? They shrink.
- Stop moving your joints? They stiffen.
- Stop stretching? Connective tissue dries out and becomes brittle.
- Stop balancing? Your brain actually downgrades those neural pathways.

And once your body decides a movement isn't necessary anymore, getting it back is a real challenge.

**The main culprits that start this process:**

- **Sedentary lifestyle**—Hours of sitting, watching TV or at the computer, driving, "taking it easy," or just not doing enough physical movement.
- **Arthritis & inflammation**—That chronic swelling that eats away at cartilage and limits your range of motion. And, most of the time, it can be traced back to a lack of activity and too many inflammatory foods.

(If you'd like my list of the top 10 anti-inflammatory foods, you can download it for free at https://aging-boldly.life/top10foods.)

- **Muscle loss**—Every decade after age 30, we naturally lose 3–8% of muscle mass, unless we fight for it. Every one of those lost muscle pounds burns around 50 calories each day just to exist. So, if you lose 10 pounds of muscle, your body is burning about 500 *fewer calories each day*. No wonder we develop a midriff bulge (and more) as we age.
- **Poor flexibility & weak connective tissue**—Tight muscles pull your joints out of alignment, and weak tendons and ligaments make every movement harder.

But here's the real kicker: when movement starts to hurt, most people **stop moving**. And that's exactly what accelerates the decline.

## The Cost of Doing Nothing

Doing nothing is the fastest way to lose your independence.

**Here's that downward spiral:**

1. **Joints stiffen and swell**—Your cartilage dries out, the joint spaces narrow, and bones start rubbing directly against each other.
2. **Muscles shrink**—Besides the reduced caloric burn, you have less strength to absorb impact, which grinds even more on your joints.

3. **Balance deteriorates**—Your reflexes slow, your stability weakens, and one stumble could mean a fracture.
4. **Mobility vanishes**—Simple tasks like getting up from the floor, carrying groceries, walking to the mailbox, or, as Camille realized, picking up keys, can become exhausting.
5. **Independence fades**—You start needing help to do the things you used to take for granted; things you used to do without thinking.

You stop moving because it hurts, and then it hurts *more* because you stop moving.

This isn't a slippery slope, *it's a freakin' landslide*!

## The No-Excuse Blueprint

1. **Stretch Daily, Gently, Intentionally.**

   Mobility is your body's WD-40. It keeps your joints gliding, blood flowing, and muscles pliable. You don't need marathon yoga sessions; just 5–10 minutes a day of targeted, gentle stretching.

   Start where you are. Do it sitting if you must. Progress is progress.

2. **Strengthen the Muscles That Support Your Joints.**

   Your muscles are the shock absorbers for your skeleton. Weaker muscles put the full brunt of every step, sit, and bend on your joints.

   Focus on the glutes, hamstrings, quads, and core. These aren't "beach muscles," they're the ones that keep you out of the nursing home.

Remember: *being strong enough to get off the toilet without help is a legitimate fitness goal!*

And, if you want a great course that covers stretching, strengthening, and much more, take a look at my **Joint Health & Mobility Course**, at https://agingboldly.life/jointhealth.

3. **Reduce Chronic Inflammation.**

   Inflammation is your body's fire alarm. It's useful in short bursts for protecting a sprained ankle or healing a cut. But it's devastating when it never shuts off. Chronic inflammation eats away at cartilage, stiffens ligaments, and erodes muscle.

   Start with food: ditch processed sugar, avoid ultra-processed junk, eat more omega-3-rich foods, and hydrate like it matters … because it does.

   Don't forget to download my free list of the top 10 anti-inflammatory foods at https://agingboldly.life/top10foods.

4. **Supplement Smart.**

   Joints don't rebuild on wishful thinking. They need raw materials—nutrients that feed cartilage, support connective tissue, and reduce inflammation.

   Sadly, due to declining soil nutrients, ultra-processing, and the prevalence of GMO products, nearly all Americans fail to meet multiple Recommended Dietary Allowances through food alone.

For example, over 90% fall short in vitamin D and E, and over 50% in magnesium; so the percentage meeting *all* RDAs through diet alone is effectively zero.

The right supplements can be the difference between slowing down the decline or reversing it.

Since nutritional supplements are such a huge and growing market, how can you determine which supplements are right for you? Which ones are actually effective?

That's where health coaches come in. I have been guiding people through the supplement maze for nearly 30 years. In a later chapter, we'll get into the weeds a bit about supplementation—the good, the bad, and the harmful. Stay tuned.

5. **Track and Celebrate.**

   When you can bend easier, walk longer, or climb stairs without thinking, write it down! Progress is the most addictive thing in the world. And once you see it, you want more of it.

   Don't wait for a "big win." Celebrate the everyday victories—every easier bend, every extra step, every pain-free morning.

## 30-Day Joint Rescue Plan—Your Daily Guide to Less Stiffness, More Strength, and Better Mobility

**Goal:** Pick one joint (knee, hip, shoulder, ankle, or spine) and commit to doing *something* for it every day for the next 30 days. Small, consistent steps win.

Ask yourself: "If I did something for this joint every day for the next 30 days, what could it feel like?"

Don't overthink it.

Don't wait for Monday.

Don't wait for "when things calm down."

Start today.

### *Daily Checklist*

**Gentle Stretching (5–10 min.)**

- Target your chosen joint first, then the muscles that support it.
- Keep it pain-free. Stretch to the point of gentle tension, never sharp pain.

**Strength Work (5–15 min.)**

- Strengthen the muscles that stabilize your joint.
- Use resistance bands, light weights, or just body weight.

**Anti-Inflammatory Habit**

- Eat at least one anti-inflammatory food daily (berries, leafy greens, salmon, olive oil, walnuts).
- Hydrate: Drink 8 to 10 glasses of water a day.
- Try to get at least 30 grams of high-quality protein at EVERY meal.
- Reduce or eliminate added sugar and highly processed foods.

**Smart Supplementation**

- Take joint-support supplements daily (glucosamine, omega-3s, collagen, etc.).
- Be consistent. Results come from regular use, not occasional bursts.

**Move More Throughout the Day**

- Walk, take the stairs, and stand up every 30 to 60 minutes.
- Movement keeps joints lubricated and muscles active.
- You can also download my **6-Minute Anywhere Workout** for free at https://agingboldly.life/workout.

**Track Your Wins**

- Write down anything that feels better: less stiffness in the morning, easier bending, longer walks, less swelling.
- Even tiny progress counts. Momentum builds on noticing change.

**Weekly Add-Ons**

- **Balance Training:** Practice standing on one leg for 20 to 30 seconds per side, two to three times a week.
- **Posture Check:** Stand tall, shoulders back, and chin up. Every time you catch yourself slouching, correct your posture.
- **Activity You Enjoy:** Participate in swimming, dancing, or tai chi—anything that keeps you moving and makes you smile.

**Three Key Takeaways**

1. Movement is not optional.
2. Movement prevents decline far better than medicine alone.
3. Nutrition and training together keep your body adaptable.

**Three Discussion Questions**

1. How flexible do you feel today compared to 10 years ago?
2. What excuses have held you back from consistent movement?
3. Where could small, daily exercises change your energy and confidence?

**Three Action Steps**

1. Schedule 10 minutes of strength or mobility work each day this week.
2. Identify one "movement excuse" you've been making and eliminate it.
3. Add one extra serving of protein to your meals daily.

Stiffness is not a sentence; it's a signal. Your body wants to move.

Your job is to listen and respond as if your independence depends on it.

Because it does.

And you've got **unfinished business.**

CHAPTER 4

# THE SHRINKING MAN AND THE EXPANDING WAISTLINE

*"Aging is not lost youth but a new stage of opportunity and strength."*

–Betty Friedan

**I'll never forget the moment.**

I was on prednisone, a corticosteroid, for 20 years for chronic asthma. I weighed 165 pounds when I started taking it. It was a powerful anti-inflammatory and the only thing that kept me out of the ER. But it came with side effects … and I got every single one.

Liver issues. Osteoporosis. And the one that shook my confidence the most: a whopping 140-pound weight gain.

There were several moments I'll never forget during that weight gain.

The first was two days before a vacation my wife and I had been looking forward to for months. I realized I had no long pants that fit, and only two shirts I could button. We were living in the Florida Keys at the time, where finding anything other than shorts and fishing shirts was hard enough—finding them in a 3X or larger? Nearly impossible.

The second moment was the first time I had to ask for a seat extender on an airline flight. I can't begin to describe the shame and embarrassment I felt in that moment. For crying out loud, I ran marathons in my 40s, and now this! Can anyone relate?

Then there were all the times I caught my reflection in a mirror. I'd have to stop and look again, because I didn't recognize the person staring back at me.

In my mind, I was still 165 pounds. But the reality was undeniable.

The muscle that used to fill my shirts was gone, replaced by a belly and pounds of fat I never remembered inviting.

I'll be honest; it really stung. Not because I was chasing my 25-year-old self, but because in that moment I realized that **this wasn't just about appearance. It was about survival.**

## The Silent Thief: Muscle Loss

As we age, we naturally lose muscle mass, a condition known as *sarcopenia*.

Starting as early as 30, you can lose 3–8% of your muscle every decade, and after 60, that rate accelerates.

But here's what most people don't realize:

- Less muscle doesn't just mean less strength; it means less balance, slower reflexes, and a higher risk of falls.
- Less muscle means fewer calories burned at rest, which means fat creeps in faster.
- Less muscle means your body has a harder time handling stress, illness, and injury.

This isn't a vanity problem; it's a functional independence problem.

It's the difference between getting off the floor and waiting for help.

Between walking across a room confidently or clinging to the furniture.

Between living life on your terms, or shrinking your world to match your limitations.

## The Real Culprits

Let's face it; muscle doesn't just "disappear." It fades because we stop challenging it.

- We sit more, lift less, and outsource physical effort.
- Most older adults don't eat enough high-quality protein to maintain or rebuild muscle.

- The myth that "lifting weights is dangerous after a certain age" keeps people weak.
- We stop moving because of discomfort, which accelerates the very weakness that caused the discomfort in the first place.

## The Dangerous Tradeout

When muscle moves out, fat usually moves in to take its place. And unlike muscle, fat just likes to hang out (literally and figuratively).

Fat is NOT metabolically helpful. It increases inflammation, stresses joints, and raises the risk for heart disease, diabetes, and cognitive decline.

Worse, the fat we gain as we age is often visceral fat, which lands in the belly, wraps around organs, and quietly undermines our health from the inside out.

## The No-Excuse Blueprint for Fighting Back

### *1. Prioritize Protein.*

You can't build muscle without the raw materials and, for most people over 60, that means aiming for at least 25–30 grams of protein per meal. I tell my clients to shoot for 30 grams or more.

Since your body can't store protein, it needs a steady supply throughout the day to build and repair cells. That might look like a protein shake for breakfast, a chicken breast or lentil soup for lunch, and salmon or lean beef for dinner.

It may sound like a lot, but even if you hit 100 grams of protein in a day, that's only about 400 calories, leaving plenty of room for healthy carbs and fats to round out a balanced diet.

**Here are some easy protein swaps:**

1. **Upgrade Your Breakfast.**
   - Instead of toast with butter → have Greek yogurt (unsweetened) with berries and a sprinkle of nuts.
   - Swap a bagel for a protein shake blended with almond milk and fruit.
2. **Boost Your Lunch.**
   - Instead of a garden salad alone → add grilled chicken, tuna, or a cup of cooked quinoa for extra protein.
   - Replace white bread in a sandwich with high-protein wraps or bread (10+ grams per serving).
3. **Power Up Snacks.**
   - Swap crackers or chips for roasted chickpeas, string cheese, or a handful of almonds.
   - Keep single-serve protein shakes or bars in your bag or car for busy days.

**Protein Reality Check** (average grams of protein per serving):

| Food Item | Serving Size | Protein (g) |
|---|---|---|
| Life Shake (I'll talk about this later) | 1 serving | 20 |
| Greek yogurt (unsweetened, nonfat) | 1 cup | 18–20 |
| Chicken breast (cooked) | 4 oz | 28 |
| Salmon | 4 oz | 26 |
| Lean ground beef (90/10) | 4 oz | 23 |
| Eggs | 2 large | 12 |
| Cottage cheese (low-fat) | 1 cup | 25 |
| Lentils (cooked) | 1 cup | 18 |
| Quinoa (cooked) | 1 cup | 8 |
| Almonds | 1 oz (about 23 nuts) | 6 |
| Peanut butter | 2 Tbsp | 7 |
| String cheese | 1 stick | 6 |
| Protein bar | 1 bar | 15–20 |

**Takeaway:**

Many "healthy" meals people eat after 60, like a salad with a few croutons or toast with jam, barely contain 5 to 8 grams of protein.

No wonder muscle is disappearing!

Hitting 30 grams of protein per meal takes *planning*, but it's easier once you know where the protein is hiding.

### 2. Lift Something ... Anything!

You don't need a gym full of equipment. Your own body weight, resistance bands, or a couple of dumbbells are enough to challenge your muscles.

The goal is progressive overload, asking your muscles to do *just a little more* over time.

### 3. Move Your Butt with Purpose.

Walking is great for your heart, but it won't stop muscle loss by itself.

Build strength days into your week and make them non-negotiable. Think squats, wall push-ups, step-ups, or band pulls.

And think about my **6-Minute Anywhere Workout** as a great starting point: https://agingboldly.life/workout

### 4. Stop Believing the Myths.

Strength training won't make you "bulky," it won't "wreck your joints," and it's *not* "just for young people."

In fact, it's the most powerful anti-aging tool you have. Strong muscles protect joints, improve balance, boost metabolism, and enhance your mood.

### 5. Feed Your Recovery.

Muscles don't grow while you're lifting; they grow while you're *resting and recovering*. Pair your workouts with quality nutrition, plenty of protein, hydration, and adequate sleep to maximize results.

**The Cost of Doing Nothing**

Do nothing, and the shrinking continues.

Your world gets smaller.

Your list of "I can't do that anymore" gets longer.

The independence you once took for granted slips away quietly.

This isn't about fear … it's about facts.

**Try This:**

Add one protein-powered habit this week:

- Have a protein shake in the morning.
- Add an extra serving of lean protein at lunch.
- Track your protein intake for the next seven days. You might be shocked at how low it is.

Here's a 7-Day Protein Challenge and a simple tracker that can help keep you on track.

7-DAY

# Protein Challenge

For the next 7 days, fuel your body with high-quality, science-backed protein from Shaklee—including NEW products that are changing the game. Track your intake below as you set a new foundation for lean muscle support, healthy aging, and long-term wellness.

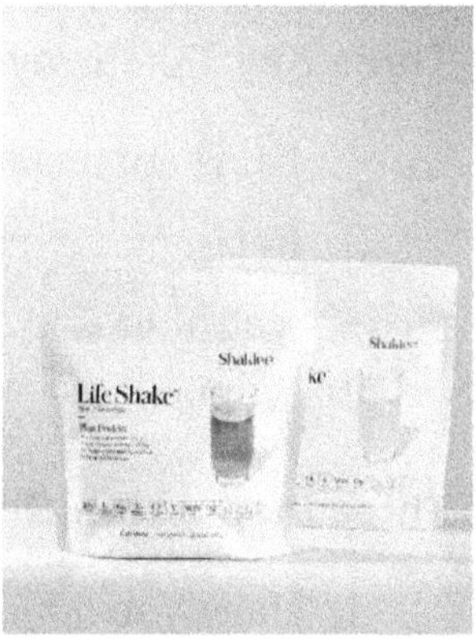


## How Much Protein Do You Need?

The general guideline for adults is:
**0.8 grams of protein per pound of body weight.**
(Ex: If you weigh 150 lbs, aim for 120 g of protein daily.)

| | DAY 1 | DAY 2 | DAY 3 | DAY 4 | DAY 5 | DAY 6 | DAY 7 |
|---|---|---|---|---|---|---|---|
| Water Intake: | ____ oz | ____ oz | ____ oz | ____ oz | ____ oz | ____ oz | ____ oz |
| Protein Goal: | ____ g | ____ g | ____ g | ____ g | ____ g | ____ g | ____ g |
| Breakfast: | ____ g | ____ g | ____ g | ____ g | ____ g | ____ g | ____ g |
| Lunch: | ____ g | ____ g | ____ g | ____ g | ____ g | ____ g | ____ g |
| Snack: | ____ g | ____ g | ____ g | ____ g | ____ g | ____ g | ____ g |
| Dinner: | ____ g | ____ g | ____ g | ____ g | ____ g | ____ g | ____ g |

## Quick Tip

Spread your protein throughout the day to support satiety, muscle building, and balanced blood sugar.

**Bonus:** Choose a simple strength move (wall push-ups, squats, resistance bands) and do 10 reps a day.

### Three Key Takeaways

1. Fat is not metabolically helpful.
2. Resistance exercise keeps us younger.
3. Nutrition and training together keep your body adaptable.

### Three Discussion Questions

1. Have you noticed changes in your strength, endurance, or body shape over the past few years? How has it affected your confidence?
2. What myths have you believed about aging and exercise?
3. How could rebuilding strength impact more than just your body … like your mood, energy, or independence?

### Three Action Steps

1. Schedule 30 minutes of strength training three times each week.
2. Find a workout buddy, either in person or virtually, to hold you accountable.
3. Have a serving of protein within 30 minutes after your workout.

Muscle is the currency of independence.

Build it back; you've got **unfinished business.**

## CHAPTER 5

# FOOD ISN'T ENOUGH ANYMORE

*"Take care of your body. It's the only place you have to live."*

–Jim Rohn

There are many people out there who believe in the power of food (I'm one of them).

Real, whole, unprocessed food.

Things you can recognize without a label: fresh vegetables, quality proteins, and healthy fats.

However, even after decades of clean eating, those same individuals are noticing disturbing changes.

They're doing everything "right": balanced, colorful, and nutrient-rich meals.

They're eating the leafy greens, the berries, the salmon. And yet …

- Their energy is dropping
- Their inflammation is increasing

- Their recovery from workouts and injuries is much slower

So, what's the problem? Sure, your body has changed with age, and that's expected. But here's the real crisis: the nutritional value of our foods has plummeted.

The fruits, vegetables, and grains we eat today contain a fraction of the vitamins and minerals they did just a few decades ago.

Over-farming, depleted soil, and modern processing have stripped our food of the very nutrients our bodies depend on for repairs, protection, and to thrive.

That means even if you're eating "healthy," you're probably still running on a nutritional deficit, leaving you more vulnerable to fatigue, illness, slower healing, and accelerated aging.

## The Turning Point

There was one moment that really drove it home. A good friend came to me after tweaking his knee during a pickleball game. Nothing major … at least it shouldn't have been.

Ten years earlier, he'd have been back to normal in a week. This time, it lingered. Every step felt like he was dragging a rock behind him.

He realized his body wasn't bouncing back the way it used to. And it wasn't just about his age; it was about what his body was missing.

That's when he became a nutrition client, as he realized he wasn't getting what he needed from his diet.

## Why Food Alone Is Rarely Enough

Here's the reality no one told us when we were younger:

- Nutrient density has dropped. Modern farming methods and depleted soil mean our fruits and vegetables simply don't have the same levels of vitamins and minerals they had 50 years ago.
- Our nutrient absorption declines as we get older. Even if you're eating well, your gut may not be absorbing the same amount of nutrients from your food as it once did.
- Life now demands more. Stress, illness, environmental toxins, and inflammation all require a higher level of nutrients than your diet alone can cover.
- Specific cellular repair needs specific nutrients. Joints, bones, muscles, and cells require specific compounds, like omega-3s, vitamin D, collagen, and antioxidants, that aren't easy to get in optimal amounts from food alone.

## From Kale to Key Nutrients

Don't get me wrong; nutrition still starts in the kitchen. But there's a point where you can't just "eat more kale" and expect to turn everything around.

The body after 60 has different needs than the body at 25:

- More protein to prevent muscle loss
- More omega-3 fatty acids to reduce inflammation

- More vitamin D, calcium, and magnesium to protect bones
- More antioxidants to fight cellular damage

When you fill those gaps strategically with supplements that are clean, clinically tested, and targeted, you give your body the raw materials it needs to rebuild, repair, and restore.

## The No-Excuse Blueprint for Smarter Supplementation

### *Step 1: Build Your Foundation.*

If you're not taking any supplements, start simple:

- High-quality multivitamin: Covers broad nutritional gaps
- Omega-3 fatty acids: Help reduce inflammation and support brain, heart, and joint health.

### *Step 2: Personalize for Your Needs.*

Already supplementing? Audit what you're taking.

- Are you getting the right form and dosage?
- Are you consistent, or are bottles sitting half-used?
- Do your supplements address your *specific* needs (joint health, mobility, bone density, energy)?

### *Step 3: Upgrade Your Quality.*

Not all supplements are created equal. Look for products that are:

- Clinically tested for purity and potency

- Backed by science (not marketing hype)
- Guaranteed for quality and results

## Discussion Questions

1. Have you ever dismissed supplements as unnecessary or "just too expensive"? What changed your mind, or what's holding you back?
2. Where in your life are you feeling the effects of nutritional gaps (energy, recovery, inflammation, etc.)?
3. What could your health look like 90 days from now if you gave your cells what they *actually need*?

## Try This (Action Step)

- If you're not taking supplements, start with a high-quality multivitamin and omega-3 fatty acids.
- If you are: Audit your supply. Upgrade what's outdated or incomplete.
- Track how you feel for 30 to 90 days (energy, recovery time, joint comfort) and notice the difference.

**Bottom line:** Food will always be the foundation. But for the aging body, targeted supplementation is the framework that will keep the whole structure standing strong.

## Why I Recommend Shaklee

I've used and trusted Shaklee products for years, not just because I've seen results in myself and my clients, but also because the quality and the science standards are unmatched.

**The Quality:**

- 100,000+ quality tests each year—far exceeding industry norms.
- Screening for 350+ contaminants—more than the U.S. Pharmacopeia standards require.
- Products are tested both in-house and by qualified third-party labs to ensure safety, purity, and potency.

**The Science:**

- **Landmark Study** (*Nutrition Journal, 2007*): Long-term Shaklee users had higher blood nutrient levels and healthier biomarkers than both single-supplement users and non-users.[1]
- **Landmark Study II** (*Current Developments in Nutrition, 2019*): Multi-supplement users (primarily Shaklee) showed a healthier pattern of cardiometabolic biomarkers compared to age-matched controls.[2]
- **Telomere Research:** Long-term Shaklee users were found to have significantly longer telomeres and a slower rate of telomere shortening compared to healthy controls.[3]

---

[1] Block G;Jensen CD;Norkus EP;Dalvi TB;Wong LG;McManus JF;Hudes ML;, "Usage Patterns, Health, and Nutritional Status of Long-Term Multiple Dietary Supplement Users: A Cross-Sectional Study," Nutrition journal, accessed September 9, 2025, https://pubmed.ncbi.nlm.nih.gov/17958896/.

[2] Sonhee Park, "Healthier Cardiometabolic Biomarkers in Shaklee 3-5 Yr Users than General US Populations," Shaklee Health Resource, March 4, 2019, https://healthresource.shaklee.com/healthier-cardiometabolic-biomarkers-shaklee-3-5-yr-users-general-us-populations/.

[3] Hong Wang et al., "Telemere Length of Multiple Dietary Supplement Users," Journal of Food & Nutrition Sciences, November 26, 2018, https://www.sciencepublishinggroup.com/article/10.11648/j.jfns.20180605.13

- **Product-Specific Data:** For example, Vivix® has been shown in a small clinical study to blunt post-meal inflammatory response when taken before a high-fat, high-carb meal.[4]

**Food vs. Supplement Reality Check** *(What you'd need to eat vs. what's in one day's supply of a Shaklee supplement):*

| Nutrient | Amount in Vitalizer/ Meology (from Shaklee) | You'd Need to Eat … |
|---|---|---|
| Vitamin D3 (2,000 IU) | 50 mcg | 20 cups fortified milk or 10 oz. wild salmon |
| Omega-3s (EPA/DHA) (900 mg) | 900 mg | 3–4 servings (4 oz. each) wild salmon |
| Vitamin C (500 mg) | 500 mg | 6 cups strawberries or 7 medium oranges |
| Calcium (600 mg) | 600 mg | 5 cups cooked broccoli or 2.5 cups yogurt |
| Magnesium (200 mg) | 200 mg | 7 cups spinach or 2 cups pumpkin seeds |
| Vitamin E (30 IU) | 20 mg | 2 cups almonds or 16 cups spinach |
| Resveratrol + Polyphenols (from Vivix®) | Equivalent to 300+ glasses of red wine | Not recommended |

[4] Ghanim H;Sia CL; Korzeniewski K; Lohano T; Abuaysheh S; Marumganti A; Chaudhuri A; Dandona P, "A Resveratrol and Polyphenol Preparation Suppresses Oxidative and Inflammatory Stress Response to a High-Fat, High-Carbohydrate Meal," The Journal of clinical endocrinology and metabolism, accessed September 9, 2025, https://pubmed.ncbi.nlm.nih.gov/21289251/.

**Why This Matters**

- Modern food simply doesn't contain the nutrient levels it once did.
- Getting everything your body needs *just* from food would require eating enormous quantities every day.
- High-quality supplements are a precise, convenient, and cost-effective way to fill those gaps.

**Bottom line:** *Not all supplements are created equal. Shaklee has the science, the quality, and the transparency to back up its claims. That's why it's the only brand I personally use and recommend.*

If you're as nerdy as I am, you'll enjoy reading all the scientific studies for yourself. Just go to https://healthresource.shaklee.com/shaklee-science.

**Three Key Takeaways**

1. Food is not just fuel — it's either medicine or poison.
2. Inflammation from poor nutrition accelerates aging.
3. Supplements can fill real gaps modern diets leave.

**Three Discussion Questions**

1. What foods make you feel sluggish, achy, or inflamed?
2. Where is your diet lacking in fresh, whole foods?
3. How do you feel about supplementation—skeptic, believer, or curious?

**Three Action Steps**

1. Replace one processed meal/snack with a whole-food option.
2. Add at least one anti-inflammatory food (like salmon, walnuts, or leafy greens) daily.
3. Meet with a trusted health coach or practitioner to evaluate your supplement needs.

**Give your body what it needs, and it will give you what you want—strength, energy, and life.**

Feed it well, because you have **unfinished business.**

## CHAPTER 6

# THE DISCIPLINE FACTOR: MOTIVATION IS FLEETING. DISCIPLINE IS FREEDOM.

*"We are what we repeatedly do. Excellence, then, is not an act, but a habit."*

–Aristotle

### Real-Life Inspiration: Joan MacDonald—From Exhausted to Empowered in Her 70s

In her early 70s, Joan MacDonald would get winded just climbing a single flight of stairs. She weighed 198 pounds and was taking medications for high blood pressure, high cholesterol, and acid reflux.

Painful arthritis and low energy had become her norm, and she was merely surviving. That is, until her daughter, Michelle, a fitness coach, delivered a blunt ultimatum: "*Make a change, or risk becoming a burden.*"

Faced with "existing, not living," Joan decided, "It's now or never."

Within weeks of her 71st birthday, Joan flew to Tulum, Mexico, to train in her daughter's "Wonder Woman" gym program. She overhauled her diet, prioritizing balanced macros across five meals a day. She started lifting weights, began drinking more water, and committed to consistent movement and better sleep.

Within a month, she had lost 10 pounds and slashed her medication in half.

Over the next five years, Joan dropped 68 pounds, reversed osteopenia, regained strength, and became a fitness influencer with more than one million followers, all while in her 70s.

Simple, repeated actions, done *even when she didn't feel like it.*

And here's the thing: discipline may not feel good at first.

But you know what feels worse? *Regret.*

## The Problem

Everyone wants the results, but few want to do what it takes to achieve them. And even fewer want to do what it takes … *consistently.*

We live in a quick-fix culture. People want "two weeks to six-pack abs" and "a shot to lose 50 pounds."

But here's the hard truth: When it comes to aging well, there are no hacks … only habits.

You don't get strong by accident.

You don't keep your mobility by luck.

And you don't preserve your independence by "winging it."

Discipline is the only force that will turn your good intentions into actual results.

## The Cost of Doing Nothing

Without discipline, small lapses become big losses:

- If you skip movement, you'll lose mobility.
- If you "forget" your protein, you'll lose muscle.
- If you stay up too late, you'll feel like crap in the morning.
- If you wing your day, you'll wonder where your health went.

The body keeps score, and it doesn't grade on a curve.

Every action you skip is like taking money from your future health bank.

Eventually, your account runs dry, and you don't get an overdraft notice.

You just have to pay the bill in the form of fatigue, pain, loss of independence, or a crisis you never saw coming.

## The No-Excuse Blueprint

### *1. Create a Morning Anchor Routine.*

Start your day with a short, predictable set of actions. Ten to 15 minutes is enough.

- Hydrate (8 to 12 oz. of water).
- Move (stretch, walk, or do a few mobility drills).
- Breathe (deep breathing or mindfulness).
- Plan your day (set one health goal).

### 2. *Decide Once, Repeat Often.*

Don't wake up and question your habits every day. It's mental quicksand. Decide once: "*I work out on Mondays, Wednesdays, and Fridays at 9 a.m.*"

Lock it in.

Build the pattern.

Kill the excuse before it starts.

### 3. *Habit Stacking (a great way to build new habits).*

Link new habits to habits you already have.

- After brushing your teeth → stretch for two minutes.
- After lunch → take your supplements.
- After dinner → prep breakfast for tomorrow.

This way, habits piggyback on things you already do automatically.

### 4. *Use Visual Cues.*

Make your habits visible and unavoidable.

- Lay out your vitamins.
- Put your workout shoes by the door.

- Keep your water bottle in sight.

What you see often, you do often.

### *5. Track the Wins.*

Humans love to see progress.

- Use a habit tracker (there's one in my Joint Health & Mobility Course) and check the boxes daily.
- Watching those boxes fill up can be incredibly motivating.

## The Challenge to You

Write this sentence down in big, bold letters:

**"My health will be the result of what I do when I don't feel like it."**

Then, pick ONE daily health habit—just one—and commit to doing it for the next seven days, no matter what.

No justifications.

No negotiations.

Just action.

### Three Key Takeaways

1. Create a daily health routine.
2. Purpose makes aging not just longer, but richer.
3. Legacy is built by intentional living now.

### Three Discussion Questions

1. What gets you out of bed with energy and excitement?
2. Who in your life benefits most when you live with purpose?
3. What unfinished business do you feel called to finish?

### Three Action Steps

1. Write your personal mission statement in one sentence.
2. Identify one activity that drains you—and one that fills you—and then adjust your week accordingly.
3. Share your mission with a trusted friend for accountability.

Remember, discipline isn't punishment; it's preparation. The stronger your habits, the longer your freedom.

When you reach the point where discipline feels automatic, that's when you realize the truth: Motivation is optional. Discipline is everything.

Develop discipline, because you have **unfinished business**.

CHAPTER 7

# WHEN THE APPLAUSE STOPS—WHO ARE YOU THEN?

*"The meaning of life is to find your gift. The purpose of life is to give it away."*

–Pablo Picasso

## The Quiet After the Curtain Falls

I spent decades stepping onto stages where the lights were hot, the music was soaring, and the applause felt like a tidal wave rolling right through me.

Every night, I knew my role.

I knew my purpose. I knew exactly who I was.

And then, one day, because of a side effect of a medication, the curtain closed … and it stayed closed.

There was no announcement. No farewell tour. No dramatic final bow. Just … quiet.

No rehearsals to prepare for. No lessons to teach. No applause waiting for me.

I had built my life around structure, discipline, and contribution, and in one quiet moment, it was gone.

Do you know what hit me harder than anything else? It was losing the *identity* that came with it.

Since this book is all about rebranding ourselves, I wanted to share this story with you.

Meet Christine Thynne. At 68, she had a career, a family, a profession—but not a performance identity. When she discovered dance classes for seniors, she joined, and she *loved* it.

Then, at 82, she premiered her very first *solo dance show* at the Edinburgh Fringe Festival! It's a defiant statement that passion and purpose don't retire with age. Discipline, courage, and curiosity keep us moving forward, and remind us that purpose isn't bound by age or applause.

## The Hidden Loss in Aging

For too many people, aging strips away the titles and roles that once defined us:

- The job you poured yourself into for decades
- The business card that opened doors
- The role of parent or caregiver that anchored your days
- The physical abilities that once made you stand out

These transitions usually don't come with a fanfare. Most of the time, they're subtle.

One day, you realize no one's asking for your advice at work anymore.

Your kids don't need you in the same way.

The phone isn't ringing with invitations or opportunities.

And without those "identities," something starts to happen: *The silent spiral.*

- We shrink—not just in activity, but in visibility, in contribution, and in self-worth.
- We start questioning our value.
- We start drifting into the background.

And before long, we're living more in memories than in the present.

## Purpose Doesn't Retire

Here's the truth most people don't want to face: Purpose isn't tied to a paycheck, a platform, or a title.

It's tied to your *impact.*

If you're still breathing, you still have something to give, something the world needs. It might look different than it did before, but it's no less important.

The danger is that too many people stop looking forward and start living backward. They keep telling the same old stories of what they *used to do,* instead of creating new ones worth telling.

## The Rallying Cry: Live Forward

You can't control every loss that comes with aging. But you *can* control whether or not you keep showing up. For example, you can:

- Mentor someone just starting out.
- Volunteer for a cause that moves you.
- Write, paint, teach, speak, or create.
- Show up for your friends, your community, and your family in new ways.

Impact isn't about scale; it's about presence. Sometimes changing just one life might be the biggest contribution you've ever made.

## The Cost of Doing Nothing

If you don't redefine your "why," you risk:

- Feeling invisible and unheard
- Slipping into apathy and isolation
- Losing the spark that gets you out of bed in the morning

Without purpose, the days begin to blur together.

Without direction, time becomes something to pass instead of something to look forward to.

## The No-Excuse Blueprint for Rediscovering Purpose

1. **Take Inventory of Your Past Roles.**

   Write down every role you've ever played: professional, personal, community-based. Then, circle the ones that made you feel most alive. This is now your new starting point.

2. **Translate Skills Into New Impact.**

   Ask yourself: *Where could my skills make a difference?* A teacher can mentor. A builder can volunteer for Habitat for Humanity. A performer can inspire through speaking or coaching.

3. **Commit to a Cause.**

   Pick one thing you care deeply about, and devote a few hours a month to it. Purpose grows with action.

4. **Create a Legacy List.**

   Write down all the contributions you still want to make in the years ahead, big or small. Put that list somewhere that you'll see it several times each day.

5. **Surround Yourself with Purpose-Seekers.**

   Your environment matters. Your circle of friends will either pull you forward or push you back. Choose the ones who refuse to let you settle.

### The Challenge to You

Finish this sentence: "I'm still here because ____________________." Find that reason that gets you out of bed in the morning.

Write it. Speak it. Post it somewhere you'll see every day.

Then take one small action this week that reflects that purpose; call someone, sign up, volunteer, share.

### *Final Word*

When your applause stops, the question isn't "Was I enough?" It's "What's next?"

Your next chapter might not be on the same stage, but it can be just as powerful. The world doesn't need your memories; it needs your *presence*.

#### Three Key Takeaways

1. Purpose doesn't retire.
2. Negative self-talk accelerates decline; possibility thinking rewires it.
3. Resilience is the secret to bouncing back more quickly.

#### Three Discussion Questions

1. What limiting belief about aging do you catch yourself repeating?

2. When was the last time you surprised yourself by learning something new?
3. Define your purpose today. What will it be a year from now?

**Three Action Steps**

1. Write down one limiting belief—then rewrite it as a possibility.
2. Learn one new skill or habit this month.
3. Practice daily gratitude for three things that prove you are still growing with purpose.

Purpose keeps you younger than any pill.

Find your purpose, because you have **unfinished business**.

CHAPTER 8

# THE COMPANY YOU KEEP—YOUR CIRCLE SHAPES YOUR FUTURE

*"You are the average of the five people you spend the most time with."*

–Jim Rohn

## The Reality Check

We like to think we're "all that": self-made, self-motivated, and immune to outside influence. But here's the uncomfortable truth: We are shaped, pulled, and often limited by the people closest to us.

Our habits, our mindset, and even our health are directly influenced by the energy, conversations, and behaviors of our inner circle. If you spend your days with people who complain, make excuses, and live in the past, you'll probably find yourself doing the same thing.

But surround yourself with people who take care of themselves, set goals, and keep learning, and you'll rise to meet their level.

You will become the sum of their habits, their mindset, and their expectations for what life will look like after 60.

If you want to age boldly, surround yourself with people who are living the way you want to live in 10 years.

The question isn't *if* the people around you are shaping you. The question is—*are they shaping you in the right direction?*

## Real-Life Inspiration: Tom Simek—Reinvention at Any Age

Tom Simek was a 59-year-old retired building contractor battling osteoporosis, high cholesterol, and sleep apnea. Overweight and unfit, he spent the majority of his days managing illness rather than regaining his strength or vibrancy. His wake-up call was a diagnosis that threatened his independence.

But Tom didn't retreat—he transformed. He started with simple daily habits:

- healthier eating
- daily walks
- bodyweight exercises

Those simple choices turned into a movement. Tom rediscovered his physicality, and 13 years later, at 72, he's competing on *American Ninja Warrior* and in the National Senior Games. He credits his new life to three healthy pillars:

1. A renewed sense of purpose every morning
2. A new social circle built through sports and training
3. Improved sleep, mobility, and mental clarity, all reinforcing one another, all built on new habits and a new community

**The Problem**

Too many of us hang on to our old circles out of habit instead of intention. We stay connected to people who:

- Reinforce our excuses
- Nurture our fears instead of challenging them
- Avoid change because it's "too much work"
- Pull the conversation backward instead of forward: a real energy suck

The older we get, the more dangerous this becomes. Because with aging, *momentum is everything*. And your circle can either fuel it … or suck the life out of it.

## The Cost of Doing Nothing

If you don't shape your inner circle with intention, you risk:

- Adopting the mindset of decline
- Matching the unhealthy habits of those around you

- Letting someone else's low expectations become your ceiling
- Losing sight of your own goals because they don't fit the group's narrative

## The No-Excuse Blueprint for Curating a Circle That Lifts You Up

1. **Take Inventory.**

   Write down the names of the five people you spend the most time with. Be honest: Do they pull you forward or push you back? When you leave their company, do you feel inspired or deflated?

2. **Add Intentionally.**

   Seek out people who are already living in the direction you want to go. If you want to stay strong, spend time with active people. If you want to continue learning, surround yourself with curious minds. If you want to stay optimistic, stay away from the constant complainers.

3. **Limit Exposure to Energy Drains.**

   You don't have to cut ties completely, but you *can* reduce the amount of time and emotional energy you give to those people who consistently bring you down.

4. **Join Purpose-Driven Communities.**

   Find spaces where the group goal aligns with your personal goals, such as a hiking group, a volunteer team, a mastermind, or an online community like Aging Mastery (https://info.agingboldly.life). When you're surrounded by people on the same mission, growth is inevitable.

5. **Be the Kind of Person You Want to Be Around.**

   Your circles aren't just about what you *get*—they're about what you *give*. Show up with the energy, positivity, and commitment you want to see in others. Leadership attracts leaders.

### The Challenge to You

Write this sentence down: "*My future will look like the lives of the people I spend the most time with.*"

Then ask yourself: Does that sentence excite me … or scare me?

If it scares you, start making changes to your inner circle *today*.

## Final Word

The right people don't just make life more enjoyable; they make success, health, and purpose *more sustainable*.

Surround yourself with people who remind you of where you're going, not just where you've been.

Because in the end, aging boldly isn't just about what you do—**it's about who you do it with.**

### Three Key Takeaways

1. Who you associate with is critical to who you become.
2. Relationships can protect health as much as exercise and diet.
3. Belonging gives life meaning at every stage.

### Three Discussion Questions

1. Do your five closest friends lift you up or bring you down?
2. Who is in your "inner circle" that supports your growth and happiness?
3. Where could you reach out and add value to someone else's life?

### Three Action Steps

1. Examine your circle of personal influence to see if changes need to be made.
2. Join one group, class, or community aligned with your values.
3. Offer encouragement or help to someone who may feel alone.

Your friends can be your ladder or your anchor.

Choose wisely, because you have **unfinished business**.

CHAPTER 9

# THE ENERGY EQUATION—MORE THAN JUST GETTING THROUGH THE DAY

*"Do not go where the path may lead, go instead where there is no path and leave a trail."*

–Ralph Waldo Emerson

## The Wake-Up Call

Have you ever felt that just "getting through the day" was the best that you could do?

You know, wake up, have coffee, get to the things that *have* to be done, and collapse at night.

Rinse. Repeat.

And maybe you thought you were just "slowing down with age." But in reality, you were running on fumes.

Over time, I've learned that low energy isn't just an inconvenience; it's a warning light. It's your body saying: *Something's off, and you need to fix it ... fast.*

## The Problem: Energy Leaks Out Everywhere

Energy is more than a good night's sleep or your morning caffeine fix. It's so much more.

Think of energy as an equation; it's your body's internal math. Just like *calories in vs. calories out* determines your weight, *energy in vs. energy out* determines how alive you feel. Every day, you're making deposits and withdrawals.

What you eat, how you move, the quality of your recovery—these are your energy deposits.

Poor nutrition, inactivity, stress load, and lack of sleep? Those are withdrawals.

Just like your checking account, when withdrawals are greater than deposits, your tank runs low. When you keep your account balanced, or even in surplus, you're not just awake, you're fully charged.

As we age, the stakes get higher. In our 20s, we all probably pulled all-nighters, skipped meals, and pushed through on fumes (especially during the college years!).

But after 60? Your body doesn't have the same ability to bounce back. Every missed meal, late night, or skipped workout takes a bigger toll, but every positive choice pays bigger dividends.

Your own Energy Equation isn't just about feeling good tomorrow; it's about having the vitality to keep living *on your terms* for decades to come. When you master your inputs and manage your energy-sucks, you don't just keep going—you keep thriving.

Here are the main ways our energy drains:

- **Poor nutrition**—not enough protein, micronutrients, or hydration
- **Inactivity**—muscles that aren't used become inefficient at producing energy.
- **Inflammation**—from processed food, stress, and unaddressed health issues
- **Mental clutter**—worry, regret, and overwhelm suck more energy than any workout.
- **Lack of recovery**—not just sleep, but real rest that lets your body and mind recharge.

The older we get, the more these energy drains matter because our body's "energy reserve tank" gets smaller.

### *The Cost of Doing Nothing*

If you ignore your energy equation:

- You wake up tired, no matter how much you sleep.
- You avoid activity because you "don't have the energy," which makes you even weaker.
- You give up opportunities, experiences, and relationships because you can't bring your best self to them.
- Worst of all, you start to believe this is "*just the way it is.*"

But the real truth is: **tired does not have to be the new normal**.

## The No-Excuse Blueprint for Energy That Lasts

1. **Feed for Fuel, Not Just Fullness.**
   - *Every meal* needs protein (25–30g), healthy fats, and fiber-rich carbs.
   - Avoid big blood sugar swings by cutting refined sugars and ultra-processed junk.
   - Hydrate; most older adults are dehydrated and mistake it for fatigue.
2. **Move to Create Energy.**
   - It sounds backward, but the more you move, the more energy your body produces.
   - Combine low-intensity movement (walking, mobility work) with strength training to build muscle. Muscle is *the ultimate energy engine*.
3. **Fight Inflammation Daily.**
   - Eat anti-inflammatory foods (salmon, walnuts, leafy greens, olive oil). You can download my Top 10 Anti-Inflammatory Food List at: agingboldly.life/Top10Foods.
   - Manage stress. Chronic stress burns through nutrients and saps your vitality.
   - Get enough sleep, and keep it consistent.
4. **Protect Your Mental Energy.**
   - Limit your time with chronic complainers and other energy-draining situations.

- Start your day with a clear plan so you're not wasting energy on constant decision-making.
- Practice gratitude. It shifts focus from what's wrong to what's possible.

5. **Supplement Smart** (see Chapter 5).
   - Fill nutrient gaps with high-quality, science-backed supplements.
   - Omega-3s, a quality multivitamin, and targeted support for inflammation and joint health can make a huge difference. Give your body what it needs, and it will serve you well.

## Real-Life Energy Makeover

Consider Jim Owen. At 70, he started with simple walks and strength training, totally changing course from a life ruled by discomfort and low energy. Fast-forward to 84: he's athletic and fully energized, winning gold in 10 events at the Senior Games. His transformation shows that real energy isn't magic; it's small, consistent, persistent work.

### The Challenge to You

This week, track your energy drains. For three days, write down:

- What you eat and drink
- How much you move
- How much (and how well) you sleep
- What situations or interactions with people leave you feeling drained

Then pick **one energy drain** and start plugging it.

Because here's the truth: **Energy is the currency of life. If you're bankrupt, you can't afford your dreams.**

### Three Key Takeaways

1. Setbacks are inevitable—quitting is optional.
2. Energy can improve your health or damage it.
3. Pain can be a teacher if you let it be.

### Three Discussion Questions

1. What has been your biggest health or life setback so far?
2. How did you respond—and what did you learn?
3. What can you do to lessen your energy drains?

### Three Action Steps

1. Write down the lesson from your hardest setback.
2. Identify one area of your life that drains your energy, and plug it.
3. Create a short phrase that reminds you: *"I can bounce back."*

Energy is the fuel that powers your purpose.

Without good energy, you can't finish your **unfinished business**.

CHAPTER 10

# THE LONGEVITY LIE—WHY JUST LIVING LONGER ISN'T THE GOAL

*"It is never too late to be what you might have been."*

–George Eliot

## The Big Misunderstanding About Aging

When most people talk about "getting older," they throw around one concept: *age expectancy*. They obsess over how many years they have left, as if more candles on the cake automatically equal a better life.

Here's the truth no one likes to admit: **Living longer doesn't matter if you're not living well.**

Who really wants to live to 100 if the last 20 years are spent in a wheelchair, staring at the ceiling, and struggling to recognize their own kids when they visit? Not me.

Of course, there are medical conditions none of us can predict or prevent. Life can throw curveballs. But here's the truth: most people give away far more control than they need to, or should.

My passion is showing you how to take that control back; to protect your mind, mobility, and independence for as long as humanly possible.

Because aging well isn't about adding more years to the end of your life; it's about packing more life into every single year you've got.

What you really want are more *healthy* years; years you can move, think clearly, travel, play with your grandkids, climb the stairs without gasping, and wake up each morning with purpose.

## The Reality Check That Hit Me

I once met a man who proudly told me he was 92. Impressive, right? But within 15 minutes, he told me about the 14 prescriptions he was on, how he couldn't walk without help, and how he spent most days watching TV because he "didn't have the energy for much else."

That conversation stuck with me. To me, that wasn't living; it was just existing.

Here was a man who had achieved *longevity*, but not *quality*.

I couldn't help thinking, *What's the point of more years if you can't use them?*

## The Longevity Lie

We've been sold the idea that aging is just about *adding time*. But what if those extra years are spent in pain, in decline, or in a chair you can't get out of without help? That's not a life—it's just an extension of survival.

**The real goal is healthspan**—the number of years you live with full function, freedom, and vitality. That's the scoreboard that matters.

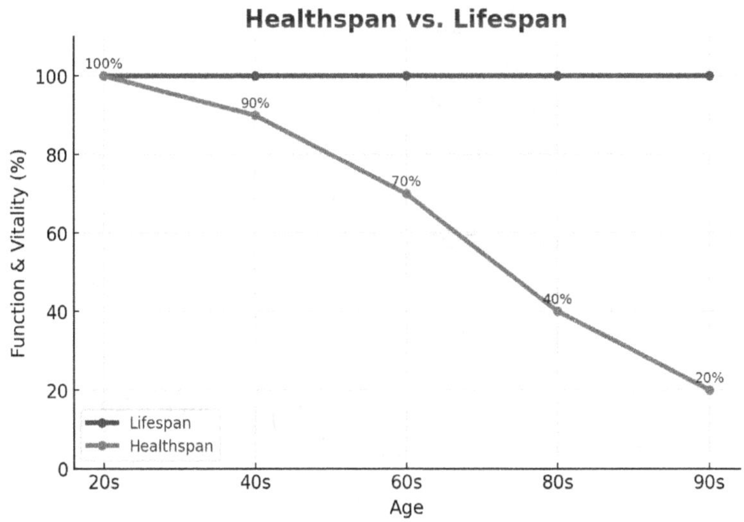


You want that green line to stay as close to the blue line as possible for as long as possible!

### *The Problem*

Too many people plan for retirement financially, but not physically. They work, save, and count the days until "freedom," only to find that their bodies can't cash the check their minds have written for all those years.

Without specific planning and action, here's what happens:

- Mobility declines faster than you expect.
- Chronic illness robs you of independence.
- Your world shrinks to match your physical limitations.

### *The Cost of Doing Nothing*

If you don't invest in your healthspan now:

- You might live longer, but spend the last decade (or two!) managing decline.
- You'll miss out on experiences that require strength, stamina, or mobility.
- You'll risk becoming dependent on others for your most basic needs.

The last thing most of us want is to be a burden. But without action, that's exactly where the path will lead.

## The No-Excuse Blueprint for Expanding Healthspan

1. **Prioritize Movement Over Mileage.**

   Forget the obsession with "10,000 steps" if those steps aren't making you stronger or more mobile. Strength training, balance work, and mobility drills will keep you independent far longer than just walking more.

2. **Eat for Function, Not Just Flavor.**

   Every bite is a deposit or a withdrawal in your future health account. Load your plate with lean protein, colorful plants, healthy fats, and anti-inflammatory foods.

3. **Protect Brain Health.**

   Challenge your mind daily. Read, learn new skills, and take up hobbies that require focus and creativity. Your brain thrives on novelty and challenge.

4. **Build Recovery Into Your Routine.**

   Quality sleep, stress management, and intentional downtime are essential for repair. A strong body without recovery is like a car losing oil; it won't last long.

5. **Get Medical Insights *Before* You Need Them.**

   Don't wait until something is wrong to get checked. Annual physicals, blood work, and proactive screenings can detect problems before they become irreversible. What you don't know can really hurt you.

## Real-Life Wake-Up Call: Ernestine Shepherd

At 56, Ernestine Shepherd had never exercised a day in her life. By the age of 70, she was a competitive bodybuilder and Guinness World Record holder as the world's oldest female bodybuilder. Now in her late 80s, she still trains six days a week, runs 10 miles regularly, and teaches fitness classes.

Her mantra? "*Age is nothing but a number, and you can start at any time.*"

She didn't just add years; she most definitely added *life* to those years.

### The Challenge to You

Write down the age you want to live to.

Now ask yourself: "How do I want to be living at that age?"

Then create a simple two-part plan:

- **Daily Action**—one thing you'll do every day to build strength, mobility, or mental clarity.
- **Weekly Action**—one thing you'll do each week to protect your healthspan (meal prep, new skill, social connection).

## Final Word

- Longevity without healthspan is just *more time to lose what you love.*
- Don't just add years to your life, add quality *life* to your years.
- The real measure of aging boldly isn't how long you're here, it's how long you can live *fully*.

### Three Key Takeaways

1. Living longer doesn't always mean living better.
2. Strength, mobility, and mental clarity can improve with the right daily actions.
3. Eat for function, not for flavor.

### Three Discussion Questions

1. What's your go-to excuse when it comes to your health?
2. What is your number one reason for wanting to increase your healthspan?
3. How often do you delay action by waiting for "perfect timing"?

### Three Action Steps

1. Write down your top excuse, and burn, shred, or delete it.
2. Tell one person your next goal, and give them permission to check on you.
3. Take one imperfect action today toward your health.

Healthspan is the difference between existing and living.

You need the best healthspan possible because you have **unfinished business**.

## CHAPTER 11

# THE MONEY MUSCLE— WHY YOUR BANK ACCOUNT MUST BE PART OF YOUR HEALTH PLAN

*"Wealth is the ability to fully experience life."*

–Henry David Thoreau

When I first started thinking seriously about my future, I thought about my health. My joints. My strength. My energy. But I wasn't thinking enough about my *financial* health until I saw what happened to friends my age who didn't plan ahead.

They weren't just cutting back on dinners out; they were making choices like skipping medications, delaying doctor visits, or staying in unhealthy relationships because they couldn't afford to leave. Their physical *independence* was all tangled up with their financial *dependence*.

That's when I realized that **money is a form of health insurance.** The more financial security you have, the more freedom you have to protect your health and live on your own terms.

### The Problem

Too many people over 60 have been sold on the idea that retirement means slowing down and living on a fixed income. But "fixed income" often really means *shrinking income*.

I remember one of my mentors, Richard Bliss Brooke, wrote in his book *The Four Year Career*, "The idea of a career has been to work (at least) 40 hours a week for 40 years (to retire) for 40% of what was never enough for that first 40 years."

Relying solely on Social Security, pensions, or savings can make you vulnerable. Inflation eats away at buying power, unexpected expenses hit hard, and before you know it, you're living a quality of life that's much lower than you planned for.

The truth is, financial stress is most definitely health stress. Money worries can raise cortisol, disrupt sleep, limit healthy food choices, and keep you from accessing care or experiences that enrich your life.

### The Cost of Doing Nothing

Without a plan for financial security, you risk:

- Running out of money before you run out of life
- Having to rely on family for financial help
- Delaying or, even worse, skipping needed medical care
- Missing out on travel, hobbies, and social opportunities
- Holding on to chronic stress that impacts your health and relationships

## The No-Excuse Blueprint for Financial Health

**Step 1: Know Your Numbers.**

Create a simple, honest snapshot of your finances: income, expenses, debt, savings, and investments. No judgment, just clarity.

**Step 2: Trim the Budget Sucks.**

Cut unnecessary recurring expenses. Negotiate bills. Cancel subscriptions you don't use. Every dollar saved is a dollar that can be redirected toward health and security.

**Step 3: Strengthen Your Income Sources.**

Multiple income sources = multiple safety nets. This is your financial "cross-training."

The key to building financial security after 60 isn't about hustling harder; it's about working smarter.

You don't need to clock 40 hours a week to create an income source that makes a difference. You just need something you enjoy that fits your lifestyle that can grow without burning you out.

That's why I'm passionate about sharing opportunities, such as my own online wellness business, which combines flexibility, purpose, and proven systems.

Because making money in your later years isn't just possible; it can be downright exciting.

- It gives you a renewed sense of purpose.
- It keeps your mind sharp.
- It pulls you into conversations, projects, and connections that light you up.
- It reminds you that you still have value to give and dreams to chase.
- It provides the resources for better health and self-care.

And the best time to start? Not "someday." Not "when things settle down." The best time is right now.

So here are 10 ideas for you to consider. (I like number 10 the best!)

### *10 Money-Making Ideas for Seniors*

1. **Freelance Skills**—Writing, editing, bookkeeping, and graphic design. Sites like Upwork and Fiverr connect you to clients.
2. **Teaching or Tutoring**—In-person or online. Share your expertise in music, art, languages, or academics.
3. **Consulting**—Turn your career experience into part-time consulting for businesses or organizations.
4. **Rent a Room or Property**—Use Airbnb or long-term rentals to monetize unused space.
5. **Pet Sitting or Dog Walking**—Low overhead, high demand.
6. **Online Store**—Sell crafts, art, vintage goods, or digital products via Etsy or Shopify.

7. **Paid Speaking or Workshops**—Teach what you know at local events, senior centers, or online webinars.
8. **Rideshare or Delivery**—If you're mobile, Uber, Lyft, and Instacart offer flexible work.
9. **Content Creation**—YouTube, blog, or podcast around your passion—eventually monetizing with ads, sponsorships, or products.
10. **Start Your Own Online Business**—Low start-up costs, flexible hours, and huge scalability. This is where my community marketing business shines; combining community, health, and income potential in one proven system.

### *A Little More About #10*

I didn't go looking for my online business. It found me at a time when I needed both better health and an extra plan for the future.

Back then, I was a professional musician, which was great for the soul, but tough on the pocketbook. I knew I wanted something that would keep me connected to people, make a real impact, and still give me the flexibility to live life on my terms.

What I found was more than a side income. It was a community of like-minded people, products that gave me better health that I believed in 100%, and a system that didn't require me to reinvent the wheel.

Over time, it became part of my way to help others transform their health while also taking control of their finances—without sacrificing their freedom.

That's why, when I talk about moneymaking ideas for seniors, this one is always at the top of my list. For me, it's not just a business; it's part of my mission.

### *Why Community Marketing Works for Older Adults*

1. **Low Risk, Low Cost**—No huge investment or long learning curve. You can start without draining your savings.
2. **Flexible Schedule**—Work when you want, where you want. Perfect for travel, caregiving, or just enjoying life.
3. **Purpose & Connection**—Stay socially engaged while helping others improve their health, finances, or lifestyle.
4. **Proven Systems**—Step-by-step training and support mean you're not starting from scratch.
5. **Scalable Income**—Start small, grow at your own pace, and create a long-term income stream.

I'm always looking for people who share my passion for helping others and creating a better life for themselves and their families.

If you'd like to learn more, you can email me directly at dean@agingboldly.life or schedule a free discovery call with me at https://meeting.agingboldly.life.

### The Challenge to You

Write down your current monthly income sources and ask yourself: *If one disappeared tomorrow, how would I replace it?*

Then choose **one** new income idea from the list above and take your first step toward making it real this week.

### Three Key Takeaways

1. Living longer requires more money.
2. There are many ways that older adults can earn additional income.
3. I still have valuable skills to use.

### Three Discussion Questions

1. Is my family financially secure for our future?
2. Do we have the funds to live the life we prepared for?
3. What additional source of income appeals to me?

### Three Action Steps

1. Take complete stock of your financial health.
2. Create your "golden years" wish list.
3. Make sure you are financially able to complete your wish list. If not, investigate one of the income sources listed.

Financial security isn't just about you; it's about what you can do and who you can lift up.

You need to be able to afford finishing your **unfinished business**.

CHAPTER 12

# YOUR TURN—PUTTING IT ALL TOGETHER

*"The longer I live, the more beautiful life becomes."*

–Frank Lloyd Wright

## From Knowing to Doing—The No-Excuse Blueprint for Aging with Purpose, Power, and Possibilities

You've read the stories. You've seen the wake-up calls. You've met the truth, sometimes in the mirror.

Now it's time to act.

Because here's the thing: reading this book will not change your life. Doing what's in this book will.

But it isn't about doing everything at once. It's about building *momentum*.

One decision.

One action.

One day at a time.

The best way to start? **Follow the blueprint.**

### ***The No-Excuse Blueprint: 12 Steps to Aging Boldly***

**Step 1: Face Your Wake-Up Call *(Chapter 1).***

Acknowledge the moment that changed everything—the fall, the diagnosis, the quiet realization that "normal" is gone. Stop wishing for the old version of you. Start creating the *next* version.

**Step 2: Refuse Invisibility *(Chapter 2).***

Visibility is a choice. Speak up. Straighten your posture. Reconnect with people. Join a group. The more you participate in life, the more life participates with you.

**Step 3: Move Every Day—No Matter What *(Chapter 3).***

Motion is life. Choose joint-friendly movement: stretching, walking, and resistance bands. Skip a day and your body notices. Skip a week and your body revolts.

**Step 4: Build Strength Like Your Independence Depends on It *(Chapter 4).***

Because it does. Aim for 30+ grams of protein per meal, and train muscles that keep you moving—legs, core, and back. This is not about looking fit. It's about staying free.

**Step 5: Fill the Nutritional Gaps *(Chapter 5).***

Food is your foundation, but it's not enough anymore. Use science-backed supplements to support immunity, joints, energy, and repair. Your cells can't run on hope.

**Step 6: Make Discipline Your Default *(Chapter 6).***

Motivation fades. Discipline stays. Anchor your habits in routines that don't require "feeling like it." The more automatic the action is, the more consistent the result.

**Step 7: Reignite Your Purpose *(Chapter 7).***

When one role ends, another purpose must be discovered. Ask: *Why am I still here?* Then do one thing every week that proves the answer.

**Step 8: Audit Your Inner Circle *(Chapter 8).***

You are the average of the five people you spend the most time with. Choose friends who lift you up, not weigh you down. Create a network of energy, not excuses.

**Step 9: Protect Your Brain *(Chapter 9).***

Cognitive decline is not inevitable. Challenge your mind daily. Learn. Create. Engage socially. Your brain is a muscle, and it responds to training.

**Step 10: Expand Your Healthspan *(Chapter 10).***

Longevity means nothing without quality. Your mission isn't to live to 100 in a wheelchair; it's to stack decades of vitality, mobility, and independence.

**Step 11: Secure Your Financial Freedom *(Chapter 11).*** Stress over money ages you faster than years. Create income sources that you control—whether it's a passion project, a side hustle, or your own business. Purpose pays.

### *Your Personal Action Plan*

Here's how to put this into motion:

1. **Pick ONE habit from Steps 3–5** and commit for 30 days.
2. **Pick ONE social connection from Steps 2, 7, or 8** and invest in it weekly.
3. **Pick ONE purpose project from Step 11** that excites you, and take the first step in 48 hours.
4. **Track your wins** daily. Success compounds when you see it.

**Bottom Line:** Aging boldly is not about doing everything. It's about doing something consistently, intentionally, and unapologetically.

**Three Key Takeaways**

1. You now have the tools—but tools unused build nothing.
2. Small, consistent steps beat big, short-lived efforts.
3. Aging boldly is not theory—it's practice.

### Three Discussion Questions

1. Which chapter hit you the hardest and why?
2. What habit or perspective shift are you most excited to start with?
3. What unfinished business will you no longer ignore?

### Three Action Steps

1. Choose one habit from this book and begin it today.
2. Create your personal "Aging Boldly Plan" for the next 90 days.
3. Share your journey with someone else because transformation multiplies when shared.

The time for learning is over.

The time for living begins now.

Time to finish your **unfinished business**.

# CHAPTER 13

# THE REST OF THE STORY

*"Age is an issue of mind over matter. If you don't mind, it doesn't matter."*

–Mark Twain

This chapter isn't about polished victories. It's about the trenches, the daily fights, the setbacks, the moments that test your spirit more than your body.

My story may look different from yours, but the ground we stand on is the same: the place where ordinary struggles forge extraordinary strength.

## A Few Incidents Along the Way

I won't drag you through the full catalog of my medical history—it would sound like I was an accident waiting to happen. But just to give you a taste:

- At nine years old, I fractured my skull … playing badminton. (Don't ask.)

- In high school wrestling, I racked up two concussions and a dislocated ankle. I'd like to say it was because I faced tough competitors, but the truth is, I just wasn't very good.
- I broke all 10 toes at once when a wave slammed a boat into them while I stood barefoot on a dock. Oy!
- Three weeks after my wife and I were married, I fell off a ladder in the Florida Keys and broke my wrist. As I lay there waiting for the ambulance, all I could think was: *Please God, don't let the fire ants get me!*

Those are just the warm-ups.

One incident, though, changed everything.

### *Facing Mortality*

I had been having some pain in my ribs for no particular reason. I had an appointment with my primary doctor, who thought it could have been caused by sleeping in an unusual position or from the jostling on a boat ride over the previous weekend. With a laugh, she tossed out, "Could be a blood clot."

We both smiled.

Six hours and one MRI later, I was being crammed into a TraumaStar helicopter and airlifted from Key West to Miami with bilateral pulmonary emboli (blood clots in both lungs)!

The pain was unbearable, but worse was the thought racing through my mind: *Am I dying?* and *I'm not ready to die!* I was literally nearly scared to death.

I put myself in the medical teams' hands, and the next morning, my attending physician delivered the "good news" with all the bedside charm of a sledgehammer: "Well, most people with those clots die within 24 hours. Looks like you might make it."

Not exactly a Hallmark moment—but I breathed a little easier.

### ***The Turning Point***

That brush with death set the stage for what came next: the accident in 2009 that truly reshaped my life. You read a glimpse of it in Chapter 1—the event that pushed me toward a new career and a mission in healthy aging.

While epic decisions sound bold, the truth is that the decisions are usually the easy part. The real fight begins the next morning, and the next … and the next.

I'd like to delve deeper into the day-to-day recovery and challenges that many of you can likely relate to in your own health journey.

That's when pain keeps dashing your hope. That's when progress feels like one step forward and five steps back.

Recovery isn't neat. It isn't quick. It isn't the glossy success story people like to imagine that makes for a good novel or movie.

It is raw. Messy. Unforgiving.

It was sweat dripping into my eyes as I strained to simply lift my legs an inch above the sheets.

It was tears no one else saw when frustration made me question my future.

It was setbacks that made me feel like I was starting over … again and again.

And it was doubt; the relentless voice asking, *Is it all worth it?*

Maybe you know what that feels like.

Maybe your battle is different—chronic pain, grief, stress, fear, or the quiet exhaustion of carrying burdens that no one else sees.

Maybe you've had mornings when even standing felt impossible, or nights when you questioned if anything would ever change.

If so, you're not alone.

So, as you read on, don't just hear *my* story—listen for the echo of your own.

Here's the truth I learned: your struggle doesn't disqualify you. It prepares you. And your next small step—no matter how shaky—could be the one that changes everything.

Here are some memories of the events that occurred during the time between the injury itself and the two years of recovery and healing that led to a new me. Looking back, a few were humorous, and I can laugh at them now.

Most weren't.

### *The Accident*

It was a Friday night in August at our home in the Florida Keys. It was hot and steamy (as always in August). My wife was out of town visiting relatives, so I decided to take my kayak out for a sunset paddle. I had done it countless times before.

But this time would be different.

The kayak was in the canal. I stepped down off the dock onto a rock ledge to climb in, but lost my balance just a bit. As I leaned to one side, the quadriceps tendons in my right leg ripped apart.

I knew the feeling; I knew the sound. I'd heard it years earlier when I tore my biceps tendon.

Down I went on the rock ledge. Friday night in August on Sugarloaf Key with no neighbors around and my wife away. *I am totally screwed!,* I thought.

I sat on that rock ledge for what seemed like an eternity, but was probably only a few minutes, trying to plan out my next move.

> **Step 1—Stand up**. I grabbed hold of the edge of the dock and managed to stand up, keeping most of my weight on my left leg.
>
> **Step 2—Get up onto the dock**. I somehow managed to get back up on the dock and stand up, again with most of my weight on my left leg.
>
> **Step 3—Get to a phone.** I realized that if I kept my right leg locked in a very stiff position, I could hobble

back toward the house. Five feet; 10 feet; 20 feet. Only a few more feet, and I could scoot backward up the 16 stairs to our front door and get to my phone!

**Step 4—It didn't happen.** Just as I approached the stairs, my right leg gave way, putting all my weight on my left leg … and the quad tendons in that leg tore apart as well. Down I went.

**Step 5—What the hell do I do now?** I couldn't move; no one was around; no phone anywhere near. I'm lying on the concrete under our stilt home, and all I could think of was that damned commercial, "*I've fallen, and I can't get up!*" I can laugh about that now, but at the time, it just wasn't that funny!

**Step 6—Get help.** Finally, after about 15 to 20 minutes, I saw a neighbor riding her bicycle in the neighborhood, and I called out. Next stop, the ambulance and the emergency room.

### *The Emergency Room*

They wheeled me into the Lower Keys Medical Center Emergency Room (and yes, we were able to get in touch with my wife), but they weren't sure what to do with me! I overheard the ER attending physician tell a nurse that he was pretty sure they'd have to amputate my right leg because the damage was so traumatic.

Thankfully, I had had a great surgeon who put my right arm back together after its tendon rupture, so I asked them to call him, and I'd wait.

Since there were not many specialists in the Keys, I was extremely lucky to have him as my surgeon. He had been the team physician for the University of Colorado football team, and had seen this injury many times before—just not in both legs at the same time!

Three days after the surgery to put my legs back together, it was time to go home. I then found out that our insurance did not cover transportation from the hospital back to our home, and neither did it cover the physical therapy I would need, especially since I was in braces from my hips to my ankles.

We decided to put the back seats down and somehow cram me into the back of my wife's Prius so I could get home to the next hurdle … those 16 steps up to the front door!

I asked the physical therapist at the hospital to teach me how to navigate steps. He wheeled me into his therapy room, and there stood the four-step practice box, which looked like Mt. Everest to me, given all that had happened.

There were handrails on the sides, so I was able to swing one leg up on a step, and then swing the other leg up to meet it—**one step at a time**. I reached the top and turned around; "Now, going down is trickier," the therapist said.

He started to describe the process, explaining how I had to be incredibly careful not to fall going down. (Really?) I looked down those four steps and remember thinking, *Screw it, I'll just go down the same way I came up—backward.*

And that's what I did—safely and securely. For the next two years, I would always go down a flight of stairs backward—**one step at a time**, which became my new mantra.

### *Recovery*

Now came the challenge. Since insurance wouldn't pay for my therapy, I hired a physical therapist to come to our home and teach me what I would need to do. We worked out a plan that I could do from the hospital bed, one that I could do with the aid of a walker, and then the long-term plan. I paid him, thanked him, and set off on my recovery journey.

My wife was working full-time, so my parents moved in with us for seven weeks to help take care of me—changing clothes, helping me bathe, changing bandages, emptying the urinal, and helping keep my spirits up.

I'll never forget the day I was finally able to get out of that bed and hobble into the bathroom on my own. It's those small, but monumental, things you remember that become milestones.

A few weeks later, I was able to resume my role as music director at Key West United Methodist Church. But first of all, I had to get there. Luckily, my parents had a Chevy Astro van, so they loaded me in there like a bundle of two-by-fours and off we went.

I remember waddling into the first choir rehearsal since the accident. There was an awkward silence, and people were unsure what to say, until Maj Johnson, my alto section leader, shouted out, “Run, Forest, run!” We all laughed, and life went on.

### *The Lesson*

There were good days and miserable days.

But here’s the only part that matters. I didn’t quit. Not because I felt strong, but because I couldn’t afford to stop. Why?

The best analogy I can think of is falling into a deep well. The walls are slick, the air is heavy, and the darkness presses in. For a moment, I think about just sitting there, waiting.

But then the truth hits me: no one even knows I’m down here.

No rope is coming.

No rescue team is on the way.

If I want out, it’s all on me. I have to figure it out for myself.

Quitting isn’t an option, because staying there means dying there.

Some days, all I had was one shaky step forward. But that step was enough. Over time, those small, stubborn choices began to add up.

They built a resilience I didn’t know I had, but desperately needed.

It’s been 16 years since that fateful August day, and I still carry some scars from it. But I also carry something else: the ability to give my clients hope, skills, and encouragement.

**2009**

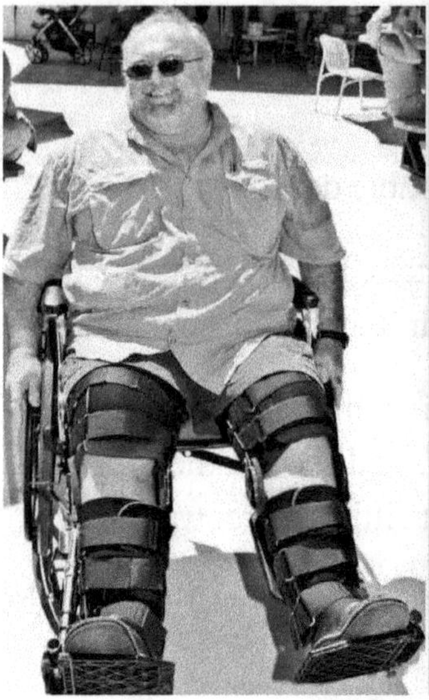

**NOW**

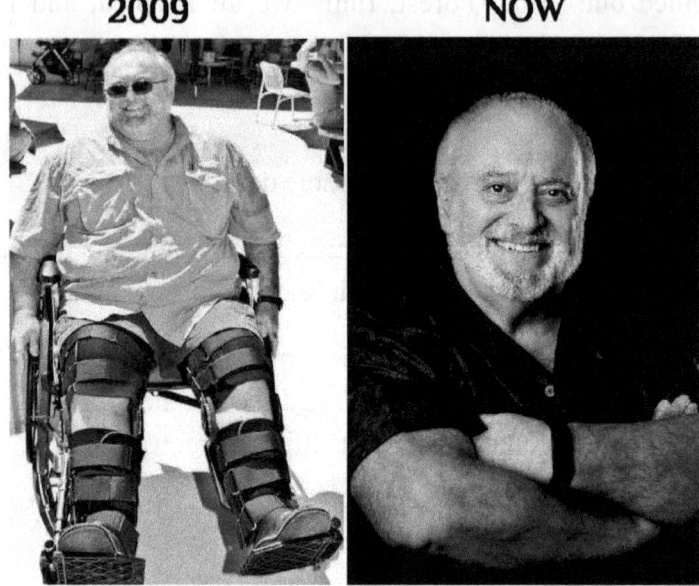

**Three Key Takeaways**

1. There are always challenges ahead.
2. It is your responsibility to be as prepared as possible for them.
3. Know who to go to for answers or find them yourself.

**Three Discussion Questions**

1. What has been your biggest health challenge?
2. What would you change in the way you dealt with it?
3. What personal unfinished health business will you no longer ignore?

**Three Action Steps**

1. Choose one new health habit to start.
2. Find an accountability partner to share your new habit with.
3. Make sure all your medical appointments and tests are up-to-date.

Healing may be messy, but it's possible.

I love this quote from Jim Rohn, "Don't wish it were easier, wish you were better. Don't wish for fewer problems, wish for more skills. Don't wish for less challenge, wish for more wisdom."

And here's my version for you:

***"Your unfinished business isn't waiting for life to get easier; it's waiting for you to decide you're not done yet."***

–Dean Walters

## CHAPTER 14

# THE FINAL CURTAIN CALL (BUT NOT THE END OF THE SHOW)

Like most of us, I've faced my share of storms. Some that I saw coming, others that blindsided me.

A curtain that came down on a career I loved.

A body reshaped by illness and medications.

A fight to regain my health and mobility.

And most recently, a cancer diagnosis.

But here's the thing … *cancer may have entered my life, but it will never be the author of my story;* and neither should anything you face.

I won't sugarcoat it; none of it has been easy. But here's the truth: every challenge has been a lesson. Every setback, a pivot point. Every obstacle, an invitation to rise again.

Cancer is just my most recent opponent. And like the others before it, I will fight with everything I have. Why? Because I'm not done yet. My story isn't over.

I have **unfinished business**, and so do you.

This entire book has been so much more than exercise plans, nutrition tips, or mindset shifts. It's been about ownership. About taking radical responsibility for your one and only body, your one and only mind, and your one and only life.

You've read the science. You've seen the strategies. You've met the people who refused to let aging steal their independence or their joy. Now, it's your turn.

Over these past chapters, you've read the hard truths and the proven strategies:

- Why movement matters, even when your joints complain
- How muscle is your best insurance policy for aging well
- Why discipline—not motivation—will save your health
- The power of purpose when the roles you've had disappear
- How nutrition, supplementation, and financial security are all part of a bigger picture

This is not theory. This is the operating manual for the rest of your life. But here's the thing—*reading it changes nothing.* Doing it changes *everything.*

Maybe you're thinking, *I'll start next month.* Or, *when things settle down.*

I get it. I've told myself those lies too.

But here's what I've learned—they're cop-outs:

- The clock isn't stopping for you to "get ready."
- Your body can't wait until you're in the mood.
- Every day you delay is a day you won't get back.

If you want to live with strength, clarity, mobility, and joy, you can't outsource that responsibility. You have to own it.

The fact that you are still here is not an accident.

If you're still breathing, you're still needed. You still have something to teach, give, build, or share.

Your next chapter isn't about chasing youth; it's about showing up for your own life so you can keep showing up for the people who matter most to you.

Because here's the most poignant truth of all: **no one is coming to do it for you**.

It's your body, your mind, your life. No one can move your body, choose your food, build your strength, or guard your energy but you.

If you wait for the "right time" to start, you'll be waiting until your opportunity has passed you by.

So, here's my challenge to you:

- Revisit the blueprint in Chapter 12.
- Pick one habit to start today. Not tomorrow … today.
- Tell someone what you're doing so they can hold you to it.

And remember, this isn't about perfection. It's about momentum. It's about stacking small, consistent wins until one day, you realize you've built a life you're proud of again.

Your purpose has not retired. Your contribution has not expired.

Every new page of your life is waiting to be written. Your struggles may shape you, but they do not own you. The decision to fight, to grow, and to live with intention is always yours to make.

I can't promise the road will be smooth. Mine certainly hasn't been. But I can promise that the effort will be worth it, because the alternative—watching life slip away while you sit on the sidelines—isn't an option for people like us.

We have **unfinished business**.

Don't waste another day watching from the sidelines. Get up, get moving, get connected, and start building the health, strength, and life you deserve.

Don't let the clock decide when you stop living. Make today the day you claim your health, your purpose, and your life back.

We all have issues. We all have scars. Your story isn't over. You have battles to fight, dreams to claim, and **unfinished business** to finish.

Start now, because the rest of your life is still yours to create.

### Three Key Takeaways

1. Don't waste another day.
2. Your body won't wait for you.
3. The effort is worth it.

### Three Discussion Questions

1. What have you been putting off?
2. How will what you've learned here change your health?
3. Who do you know that needs this?

### Three Action Steps

1. Start your plan today.
2. Track your progress proudly.
3. Share your journey with someone else because transformation multiplies when shared.

We all have **unfinished business**, and the world is waiting for us to finish it.

## Three Key Takeaways

[illegible]

# YOUR NEXT STEPS

If you have found this book helpful—if it has been the wake-up call, the nudge, or even the butt-kick you've needed—please don't keep it to yourself. Share it with someone you care about. Someone you'd want walking beside you in the years ahead.

## Stay Connected

- Visit my website: agingboldly.life
- Email me directly: dean@agingboldly.life
- For **speaking engagement inquiries**, please email me at the same address.

## Join the Community

- Be part of my **Aging Mastery Membership Group**: info.agingboldly.life

## Free Resources

- **6-Minute Anywhere Workout**: agingboldly.life/workout
- **Top 10 Anti-Inflammatory Foods List**: agingboldly.life/top10foods

## Courses & Coaching

- Explore my **Joint Health & Mobility Course**: aging-boldly.life/jointhealth
- To work with me privately, book your **Free 30-Minute Consultation** at: meeting.agingboldly.life

## Nutrition & Wellness

- Shop my **Nutritional Storefront** for proven, science-based products: nutrition.agingboldly.life

And please, share your own story with me at dean@aging-boldly.life. I want to know where you've been, what you're facing, and where you're determined to go.

Let's finish our **unfinished business** together.

# MORE QUOTES ON AGING

May these words bring you wisdom, laughter, and inspiration. Some are short and sweet, others tell a story, and a few will make you stop and think. Each one carries a truth worth holding onto.

- "The longer I live, the more beautiful life becomes." ~Frank Lloyd Wright
- "There is a fountain of youth: it is your mind, your talents, the creativity you bring to your life and the lives of people you love. When you learn to tap this source, you will truly have defeated age." ~Sophia Loren
- "In the central place of every heart, there is a recording chamber. So long as it receives a message of beauty, hope, cheer, and courage—so long are you young. When the wires are all down and our heart is covered with the snow of pessimism and the ice of cynicism, then, and only then, are you grown old." ~Douglas MacArthur
- "For the unlearned, old age is winter; for the learned, it is the season of the harvest." ~Hasidic saying
- "Every year should teach you something valuable; whether you get the lesson is up to you. Every year

brings you closer to expressing your whole and healed self." ~Oprah Winfrey

- "One of the reasons people get old—lose their aliveness—is that they get weighed down by all of their stuff." ~Richard Leider
- "I suppose real old age begins when one looks backward rather than forward." ~Mary Sarton
- "Of all the self-fulfilling prophecies in our culture, the assumption that aging means decline and poor health is probably the deadliest." ~Marilyn Ferguson
- "Age is no barrier. It's a limitation you put on your mind." ~Jackie Joyner-Kersee
- "Your 40s are good. Your 50s are great. Your 60s are fab. And 70 is f*@king awesome!" ~Helen Mirren
- "Know that you are the perfect age. Each year is special and precious, for you shall only live it once. Be comfortable with growing older." ~Louise Hay
- "Oh, the worst of all tragedies is not to die young, but to live until I am seventy-five and yet not ever truly to have lived." ~Martin Luther King Jr.
- "You don't stop laughing when you grow old, you grow old when you stop laughing." ~George Bernard Shaw
- "I believe the second half of one's life is meant to be better than the first half. The first half is finding out how you do it. And the second half is enjoying it." ~Frances Lear

- "We are not victims of aging, sickness, and death. These are part of scenery, not the seer, who is immune to any form of change. This seer is the spirit, the expression of eternal being." ~Deepak Chopra
- "Anyone who keeps the ability to see beauty never grows old." ~Franz Kafka
- "To find joy in work is to discover the fountain of youth." ~Pearl S. Buck
- "The trouble is, when a number—your age—becomes your identity, you've given away your power to choose your future." ~Richard J. Leider
- "It annoys me when people say, 'Even if you're old, you can be young at heart!' Hiding inside this well-meaning phrase is a deep cultural assumption that old is bad and young is good. What's wrong with being old at heart, I'd like to know? Wouldn't you like to be loved by people whose hearts have practiced loving for a long time?" ~Susan Moon
- "I've always said that I will never let an old person into my body. That is, I don't believe in 'thinking' old. Don't program yourself to break down as you age with thoughts that decline is inevitable." ~Wayne Dyer
- "Old age is an excellent time for outrage. My goal is to say or do at least one outrageous thing every week." ~Maggie Kuhn
- "A human being would certainly not grow to be 70 or 80 years old if this longevity had no meaning for the

species to which he belongs. The afternoon of human life must also have a significance of its own and cannot be merely a pitiful appendage to life's morning." ~Carl Jung

- "The belief that youth is the happiest time of life is founded on a fallacy. The happiest person is the person who thinks the most interesting thoughts, and we grow happier as we grow older." ~William Lyon Phelps
- "Getting old is like climbing a mountain; you get a little out of breath, but the view is much better!" ~Ingrid Bergman
- "If you associate enough with older people who do enjoy their lives, who are not stored away in any golden ghettos, you will gain a sense of continuity and of the possibility for a full life." ~Margaret Mead
- "When it comes to staying young, a mind-lift beats a face-lift any day." ~Marty Bucella
- "My physical body may be less efficient and less beautiful in old age. But God has given me an enormous compensation: my mind is richer, my soul is broader, and my wisdom is at a peak. I am so happy with the riches of my advanced peak age that, contrary to Faust, I would not wish to return to youth." ~Robert Muller
- "None are so old as those who have outlived enthusiasm." ~Henry David Thoreau
- "Elderly people are like plants. Whereas some go to seed, or to pot, others blossom in the most wonderful ways. I believe beauty competitions should be held

only for people over seventy years of age. When we are young, we have the face and figure God gave us. We did nothing to earn our good looks. But as we get older, character becomes etched on our face. Beautiful old people are works of art. Like a white candle in a holy place, so is the beauty of an aged face." ~James Simpson

- "I'm baffled that anyone might not think women get more beautiful as they get older. Confidence comes with age, and looking beautiful comes from the confidence someone has in themselves." ~Kate Winslet
- "The wiser mind mourns less for what age takes away than what it leaves behind." ~William Wordsworth
- "Grow old along with me! The best is yet to be." ~Robert Browning
- "Aging is not lost youth but a new stage of opportunity and strength." ~Betty Friedan
- "Anyone who stops learning is old, whether at twenty or eighty. Anyone who keeps learning stays young. The greatest thing in life is to keep your mind young." ~Henry Ford
- "Here's what I know: I'm a better person at fifty than I was at forty-eight … and better at fifty-two than I was at fifty. I'm calmer, easier to live with. All this stuff is in my soul forever. Just don't get lazy. Work at your relationships all the time. Take care of friendships, hold people you love close to you, take advantage of birthdays to celebrate fiercely. It's the worrying—not

the years themselves—that will make you less of a woman." ~Patti LaBelle

- "Relish love in our old age! Aged love is like aged wine; it becomes more satisfying, more refreshing, more valuable, more appreciated, and more intoxicating." ~Leo Buscaglia
- "Getting old is a fascination thing. The older you get, the older you want to get." ~Keith Richards
- "In the end, it's not the years in your life that count. It's the life in your years." ~Abraham Lincoln
- "Count your age by friends, not years. Count your life by smiles, not tears." ~John Lennon
- "I am appalled that the term we use to talk about aging is 'anti.' Aging is as natural as a baby's softness and scent. Aging is human evolution in its pure form." ~Jamie Lee Curtis
- "Do not grow old, no matter how long you live. Never cease to stand like curious children before the great mystery into which we were born." ~Albert Einstein
- "Aging isn't about getting old, it's about LIVING … Learning that you can age well will actually help you to age better … let's start celebrating and living an engaged life, and stop punishing ourselves for not looking a certain way, and instead holding ourselves accountable for actually taking care of ourselves inside first, knowing the results on the exterior will be a shining side effect." ~Cameron Diaz

- "In spite of illness, in spite even of the archenemy sorrow, one can remain alive long past the usual date of disintegration if one is unafraid of change, insatiable in intellectual curiosity, interested in big things, and happy in small ways." ~Edith Wharton
- "I have absolutely no objection to growing older. I am a stroke survivor, so I am extremely grateful to be aging—I have nothing but gratitude for the passing years. I am aging—lucky, lucky me!" ~Sharon Stone
- "It's like you trade the virility of the body for the agility of the spirit." ~Elizabeth Lesser
- "I love living. I love that I'm alive to love my age. There are many people who went to bed just as I did yesterday evening and didn't wake this morning. I love and feel very blessed that I did." ~Maya Angelou
- "Aging happy and well, instead of sad and sick, is at least under some personal control. We have considerable control over our weight, our exercise, our education, and our abuse of cigarettes and alcohol. With hard work and/or therapy, our relationships with our spouses and our coping styles can be changed for the better. A successful old age may lie not so much in our stars and genes as in ourselves." ~George E. Vaillant
- "I don't believe in aging. I believe in forever altering one's aspect to the sun." ~Virginia Woolf
- "With age comes the inner, the higher life. Who would be forever young, to dwell always in externals?" ~Elizabeth Cady Stanton

- "The great thing about getting older is that you become more mellow. Things aren't as black and white, and you become much more tolerant. You can see the good in things much more easily rather than getting enraged as you used to do when you were young." ~Maeve Binchy
- "We don't grow older, we grow riper." ~Pablo Picasso
- "Beautiful young people are accidents of nature, but beautiful old people are works of art." ~Eleanor Roosevelt
- "Those who love deeply never grow old; they may die of old age, but they die young." ~Benjamin Franklin
- "Aging is an inevitable process. I surely wouldn't want to grow younger. The older you become, the more you know; your bank account of knowledge is much richer." ~William Holden
- "Aging is not lost youth but a new stage of opportunity and strength." ~Betty Friedan
- "We don't stop playing because we grow old; we grow old because we stop playing." ~George Bernard Shaw
- "The great secret that all old people share is that you really haven't changed in 70 or 80 years. Your body changes, but you don't change at all." ~Doris Lessing
- "In fact, looking back, it seems to me that I was clueless until I was about 50 years old." ~Nora Ephron
- "I have reached the age when, if someone tells me to wear socks, I don't have to." ~Albert Einstein

You have **unfinished business**.

# MORE INSPIRING STORIES

## The Power of a Late Start

Most people think that life's biggest opportunities pass us by once we hit 60 (or even 50!). That's a lie.

The truth is, the years after 60 can be the most powerful, creative, and productive decades, if you decide they will be.

You've got wisdom you couldn't buy in your 20s, experience you couldn't fake in your 30s, and (if you play your cards right) the energy to put them both to work.

The following stories aren't just about "successful" people. They're about ordinary people who refused to accept the idea that their best years were behind them.

They started new careers in all walks of life, built global brands, broke world records, and inspired millions … *all after the age when most people are thinking about winding down.*

And yes, you'll even see the story of Dr. Forrest C. Shaklee, the man who built a health empire in his 60s, and whose legacy is a 70-year-old company that continues to change my life, and the lives of millions of people worldwide.

Read these stories, and one thing will become very clear: you can start right now, at whatever age you are, and completely change the rest of your life.

**Colonel Harland Sanders**

By 65, Harland Sanders had endured more failures than most people could stomach: failed businesses, lost jobs, and even being pushed out of his own restaurant when the highway changed traffic patterns. Most people would have quit.

But with nothing more than a fried chicken recipe, a handshake, and a dream, Sanders traveled the country, cooking for restaurant owners and offering them a franchise deal. He slept in his car, faced rejection after rejection, and kept going until someone said "yes."

Within a decade, Kentucky Fried Chicken was a global phenomenon, and Sanders (white suit, black string tie, and all) became one of the most recognizable figures in business. His story is proof that one big idea and relentless persistence can completely rewrite your life's story.

**Laura Ingalls Wilder**

Laura Wilder spent most of her life as a farmer's wife, raising her daughter and occasionally writing short pieces for local papers. It wasn't until her 60s that she decided to tell her life story, the tale of growing up on the American frontier.

Her first book, *Little House in the Big Woods*, was published when she was 65. It became the start of the *Little House* series, which would sell millions of copies, be translated into dozens of languages, and inspire a beloved TV show.

Wilder's work didn't just entertain; it preserved a piece of American history. She showed the world that decades of life experience can be the richest source of creativity.

**Ray Kroc**

For decades, Ray Kroc sold milkshake machines, scraping by with a modest income. At 52, he walked into a small California burger stand owned by the McDonald brothers, and saw a gold mine where others saw a local diner.

Kroc convinced them to let him franchise the brand. By 59, he bought them out and built McDonald's into a fast-food empire with thousands of locations worldwide. His drive, vision, and no-quit attitude turned a local operation into a global powerhouse.

Kroc's late-blooming success shows that spotting an opportunity and acting decisively can change everything, even if your first 50 years were unremarkable.

**Anna Mary Robertson "Grandma" Moses**

A farmer's wife and mother of 10, Grandma Moses didn't pick up a paintbrush until her late 70s. For decades, she had embroidered scenes of rural life, but arthritis made stitching too painful. So, she turned to painting on cardboard, wood, and canvas.

Her work was full of charm and nostalgia and caught the attention of collectors. By her 80s, she was one of the most famous painters in America. Her art was displayed in museums and reproduced on greeting cards, calendars, and books.

Grandma Moses' story reminds us that creativity knows no expiration date. And sometimes, the thing you're "meant to do" waits patiently until you're ready for it.

**Peter Roget**

Peter Roget had a long career as a doctor, lecturer, and scientist. But the work that made his name known around the world didn't begin until he was in his 60s.

Roget had been making lists of words since childhood, a habit he used to fight depression and keep his mind sharp.

In his retirement, he decided to organize and publish them. At 73, he released *Roget's Thesaurus of English Words and Phrases*, a tool that revolutionized writing and communication.

More than 170 years later, writers still rely on Roget's work daily. His example shows that the things we do for ourselves—our hobbies, quirks, and private passions—might one day become our legacy.

**Harriette Thompson**

A concert pianist for decades, Harriette Thompson didn't run her first marathon until she was 76. Most people thought it was a charming "bucket list" item. But she kept going, year after year.

At 92, she became the oldest woman ever to finish a marathon, running the 26.2-mile course despite battling cancer. Her determination and courage became a global inspiration, showing that resilience matters more than perfect health.

Thompson's example reminds us: it's not too late to start, and it's never too late to keep going.

**Diana Nyad**

Diana Nyad was a champion swimmer in her youth, but her greatest triumph came at 64. After four failed attempts, she finally swam from Cuba to Florida without a shark cage: 110 grueling miles through jellyfish-filled, stormy waters.

She endured extreme exhaustion, swelling, and stings, but kept repeating her mantra: *Find a way.* When she stepped onto the Florida shore, she became a symbol of unshakable perseverance.

I lived in the Keys at that time and was fortunate enough to be on the shoreline (with hundreds of others) when Diana Nyad came ashore that day, September 2, 2013. Being there at that precise historical moment was an experience I'll never forget.

Nyad's story is a reminder that unfinished dreams don't expire; they wait for you to chase them again.

**Vera Wang**

Vera Wang's path to fashion stardom was anything but straight. A competitive figure skater turned journalist, she didn't design her first dress until she was 40. But it was in her 50s and beyond that her name became synonymous with luxury bridal fashion.

Her signature style, blending classic elegance with modern flair, transformed the industry. Today, her brand spans clothing, fragrances, jewelry, and home décor—proof that reinvention is possible at any age.

Wang's career shows that your earlier skills, even from unrelated fields, can fuel a second act that eclipses the first.

### Dr. Forrest C. Shaklee

Born in 1894, Forrest C. Shaklee's early life was marked by hardship. Diagnosed with tuberculosis as a child, doctors predicted he wouldn't live long. Instead of accepting that fate, he took control of his health, studying nutrition, the human body, and the power of natural remedies long before "wellness" became a buzzword.

By 1915, he had become a chiropractor and nutritionist, pioneering holistic health principles that would influence generations to come. But his biggest move came much later, when, in 1956, at the age of 62, he founded the Shaklee Corporation.

He created the first multivitamin in the U.S., built an entire line of natural health products, and laid the foundation for the wellness industry we know today.

Dr. Shaklee proved that age is no barrier to innovation. His philosophy was simple: "The best way to predict the future is to create it."

He didn't just live that philosophy; he built an empire on it. And I'm proud to help carry on his legacy.

## Your Turn

If these stories prove anything, it's that time is not your enemy. *Wasted time is.*

Every single one of these people could have believed the lie that they were "too old" to try something new. They didn't.

They acted, and the second half of their lives became their best half.

Your age is not the finish line; it's just the next lap. Whether you want to start a business, write a book, transform your health, or pursue a lifelong dream, there is no better time than right now. The people you just read about started with the same 24 hours in a day that you have.

The only question left is: What will you do with yours?

You have **unfinished business**.

# ACKNOWLEDGMENTS

To my wife, Sandy, my life partner in health, purpose, and everything in between, thank you for believing in me even when I forgot how. Thank you for helping me through each injury, each surgery, each recovery, each challenge. I know I said in our vows, "I promise it will never be dull," and I was right!

To my family, my parents, and my sister, who always supported me, even though they didn't always understand my path.

To my daughter, Lina Lindenblad, who entered my life when she was 14, and has blessed me with a daughter's love and two beautiful grandchildren, Lily and Ella. Now I can witness what happens in those first 14 years!

To my best friend, Philip Salter, who was the best man at my wedding and witnessed all the events of my life that have transpired.

To the clients, colleagues, and friends who've trusted me with your wellness journeys, you've taught me more than I've ever taught you.

To my Aging Boldly community, you are living proof that strength, energy, and passion don't retire. They evolve.

To my Shaklee family who have mentored me over the last 28+ years, thank you for helping me turn purpose into a mission: Dr. K. Sow, Roland Oosterhouse, Carolyn Wightman, Barb & Ray Madorin, Jennifer Glacken, Jan Hurley, and Jeannie Weiss.

To those who taught and inspired me (even though they may not know it): Eric Worre, Richard Bliss Brooke, Kristin Hall, Helen Martin, Michelle Cunningham, Sarah Robbins, and Dr. Tonya Hartig.

And finally, to the old version of me, the one who didn't give in. Thank you for getting through the hardest parts; for doing what you could, even when it didn't feel like enough; for not giving up, even when it felt like things were slipping away.

You didn't stay down.

And that made all the difference, because I've got **unfinished business.**

# ABOUT THE AUTHOR

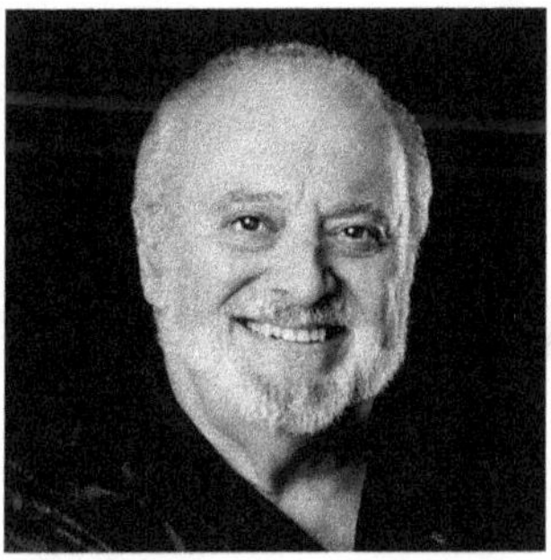

Dean Walters is a certified health coach, personal trainer, motivational speaker, and lifelong teacher who helps older adults reclaim strength, vitality, and purpose. A former opera singer, voice teacher, and conductor, Dean now channels his passion for performance into helping others age boldly through movement, mindset, and mission.

As the founder of *Aging Boldly* and the *Aging Mastery* community, he empowers people to stop coasting and start thriving. He lives in Fort Myers, Florida, with his wife, and can often be found lifting weights, leading health challenges, prepping for his next 20-mile hike, or relaxing in his garage workshop.

## Training and Certifications

Certified Integrative Nutrition Health Coach (IIN)

International Sports Sciences Association (ISSA) Certifications:

- Senior Fitness Specialist
- Fitness Nutrition Specialist

- Corrective Exercise Specialist
- Weight Management Specialist
- Bodybuilding Specialist
- Glute Specialist

Specialty training in:

- Exercise for Knee & Hip Replacement
- Shoulder Girdle Stabilization
- Parkinson's Disease
- Exercise for Breast Cancer Survivors
- Group Exercise and Physiology of Obesity

Member of the American Association of Drugless Practitioners

www.ingramcontent.com/pod-product-compliance
Lightning Source LLC
Chambersburg PA
CBHW060506030426
42337CB00015B/1762
* 9 7 9 8 9 9 3 1 6 6 2 6 1 *